The Political Economy of Organ Transplantation

This innovative work combines a rigorous academic analysis of the political economy of organ supply for transplantation with autobiographical narratives that illuminate the complex experience of being an organ recipient.

Organs for transplantations come from two sources: living or postmortem organ donations. These sources set different routes of movement from one body to another. Postmortem organ donations are mainly sourced and allocated by state agencies, while living organ donations are the result of informal relations between donor and recipient. Each route traverses different social institutions, determines discrete interaction between donor and recipient, and is charged with moral meanings that can be competing and contrasting. The political economy of organs for transplants is the gamut of these routes and their interconnections, and this book suggests how such a political economy looks like: what are its features and contours, its negotiation of the roles of the state, market, and the family in procuring organs for transplantations, and its ultimate moral justifications. Drawing on Boas' personal experiences of waiting, searching, and obtaining organs, each autobiographical section of the book sheds light on a different aspect of the discussed political economy of organs – postmortem donations, parental donation, and organ market – and illustrates the experience of living with the fear of rejection and the intimidation of chronic shortage.

A *Political Economy of Organ Transplantation* is of interest to students and academics with an interest in bioethics, sociology of health and illness, medical anthropology, and science and technology studies.

Hagai Boas is a sociologist of health and an organ recipient. He is positioned as the director of the science, technology, and society unit at Van Leer Jerusalem Institute and is an adjunct senior lecturer at Ben Gurion University of the Negev. His fields of interest include the sociology of transplant medicine and bioethics.

Routledge Studies in the Sociology of Health and Illness

For more information about this series, please visit: https://www.routledge.com/Routledge-Studies-in-the-Sociology-of-Health-and-Illness/book-series/RSSHI

The Political Economy of Organ Transplantation

Where Do Organs Come From?

Hagai Boas

Routledge
Taylor & Francis Group

LONDON AND NEW YORK

First published 2023
by Routledge
4 Park Square, Milton Park, Abingdon, Oxon OX14 4RN

and by Routledge
605 Third Avenue, New York, NY 10158

Routledge is an imprint of the Taylor & Francis Group, an informa business

© 2023 **Hagai Boas**

British Library Cataloguing-in-Publication Data
A catalogue record for this book is available from the British Library

Library of Congress Cataloging-in-Publication Data
A catalog record has been requested for this book

ISBN: 978-1-032-26567-4 (hbk)
ISBN: 978-1-032-33111-9 (pbk)
ISBN: 978-1-003-28888-6 (ebk)

DOI: 10.4324/9781003288886

Typeset in Goudy
by codeMantra

To my family

Contents

Figures and Tables

Preface

Writing about organ transplants is hard for me. Too often, I've thought about the transplant as a drama that started and ended. A medical complication I encountered and from which I recovered thanks to others. A story that is behind me. I could rather easily disappear in the crowd and continue my trivial life. Without a fistula for dialysis treatments, without severe dietary restrictions, and without too-frequent visits to the hospital, my life as a kidney recipient, so I hoped, would be just another aspect – albeit a very central and personal one – in my array of identities. It wasn't a secret, but it also wasn't something I told everyone. For the environment in which I grew up, my schoolmates, my distant relatives, it was a kind of curiosity, an interesting topic, perhaps a bit of gossip – just as transplantation medicine was considered in general: a kind of medical wonder, an interesting topic to discuss and think about, a good story for a magazine, and a personal interest story.

And, indeed, the public does take an interest in the sensation of the technology of organ transplantation: the transfer of an organ from one body to another, breaching the line that separates me from the other, between the life of the living organ and the dead body of the donor, a symbol of sacrifice and altruism. Reality, of course, is more complicated and far from the images and metaphors that the public's imagination ascribes to transplantation. My first level of difficulty in writing about transplantation derives precisely from this discrepancy, between the expectation of yet another narrative of suffering and rescue, awe, and amazement. No one likes to be a butterfly on a pin in an exhibition of social exoticism, and perhaps it is preferable to hide and not to dance to a tune known in advance.

That was my life strategy after the first transplant I underwent at age 13. It held up until the trauma of the second transplant at age 26. Then, I understood that being a young transplant patient could not remain an event you leave behind. It is a continuing experience that dictates the course of your life. And yet – how many transplant recipients are there? Worldwide they're just a minuscule fraction. Perhaps we could populate a mid-sized city. Not more. That is precisely the tragedy at the heart of this book: The shortage of organs makes it impossible for many of those waiting for a transplant to enjoy the healthy life that this technology can grant. Why are the lives of those waiting for transplants interesting at all, other than just another item on the menu of our medical anxieties?

After my second transplant, I understood that the story of organ transplantations is greater than the sum of its parts. True, we are not many, and we are far from what demographers call "a trend" or "a pattern," but the great interest that transplantation medicine attracts is related to the challenge that it poses to the fundamental forms of life in modern society. The very fact, clear and decisive, that one's life is a direct outcome of someone else's action, that one's life and fate depend on another, is a truth that, surprisingly, is not readily apparent. True, we are all here thanks to others. One's entire life is but a tangled web of connections with those near and far. Our individual lives depend on others and the social world is part of our lives more than we are willing to admit. The homes in which we live, the sidewalks on which we walk, the food we eat, even our most intimate choices – all are but steps along pathways that others have paved for us. Nevertheless, we prefer to tell the story of our lives in the first person singular. We appropriate as our own and as the outcome of our efforts all our achievements, failures, opinions, beliefs, thoughts, love, and imaginations; they are ours for better or worse. We are different from each other, and this difference we ascribe to our uniqueness – the ethos of the self as totally unique.

The tension between the perception of the self as independent and the dependence on others is perhaps the great irony of the social reality of the modern era. It is difficult to think of a work of sociology that does not deal in one way or another with an aspect of this internal irony regarding the life of the individual in the era of the masses. In this respect, organ transplants are an additional link in the effort to decipher the meaning of the contradiction between "man in society and society in man," as sociologist Peter Berger put it.

That is my second difficulty in writing about transplantation. Every piece written about transplants is about couples: Me and my donor, me and the family that donated its son's organs, me and the guy who sold his organs, me and my family. For transplant recipients, the matter of dependence on others can't be denied. When I write about organ transplants I'm writing not only about myself. I'm writing but also where I got the organs that were transplanted into me. The life of every transplant recipient is actually an answer to the question of where organs come from. Therefore, every reflection about myself as a transplant recipient and every story of transplantation and coping with it is actually a reflection on the social story of the organ economy. It's never the story of a single heroic individual. It's always a shared story.

Whereas the idea of the difference that distinguishes us is the basis for each of us imagining ourself as the star of the movie of our life, for those in need of transplantation medicine, the dependence on others is the main plot line. Thus, difference and dependence become central concepts in the everyday lives of those awaiting an organ, in the organ's acceptance, and in the constant struggle against its rejection.

Can these internal experiences and this individual understanding of self-management be turned into an insight in the social sciences? There are no organ transplants without organs for transplantation. The life of an individual depends on the life of the other; the body of one becomes part of the body of another.

In other words, every understanding regarding transplantation medicine is an exercise in sociology. Like social thinking, transplantation medicine is built on the tension between dependence and difference. It is built upon the correct interpretation of the question of the boundary between the self and the other and between the individual and the social.

This is a counter-intuitive insight because we are living in an era that celebrates individual heroism, the effort the individual invests in building his or her world and singularity, and the individualism and uniqueness that define each one of us. Therefore, I found it particularly difficult to write about transplantation medicine, certainly in the first person. This is not a personal book. Organ transplants are always the story of more than one person. The earlier version of the book, which appeared in Hebrew, was titled *The Plural Me*.

And yet, until now – until very recently – it was considered a curiosity: the individual who was actually plural. A sub-genre, perhaps, of fictional social science. But 2020 changed the picture. The COVID-19 pandemic gave birth to the concept of the "new normal" and the directive "living with" and primarily led individuals to give up the illusion of uniqueness and understand the probability that their lives are connected to those of others, exactly like those of organ recipients.

At the start of the pandemic, when there was no vaccine or medicine, the feeling of endangerment burst forth and became part of every aspect of life. The reality of the health risk took on a new shape. Health was no longer a matter for the individual or of individual responsibility – eating correctly, maintaining physical fitness, living correctly – but instead became a social question. Health in the era of COVID-19 demonstrated our dependence on the behavior of those around us: Do they maintain a social distance, do they wear a mask, do they quarantine, if verified? The extent to which the health of each one of us was the derivative of the health of all, of others, became crystal clear. Without a vaccine or a medicine for the virus, everyone suddenly became vulnerable.

The citizens of the world of plenty in the global north and west lost their confident omnipotence. From the collective subconscious arose the specter of the collapse of the civilized order, of streets empty of human beings, of businesses failing, of continuing quarantines and lockdowns, some of them – as in Melbourne – lasting months. Thus, the COVID-19 crisis joined a series of threats and dangers that shook up the social order that was consolidated at the end of the previous century and governed by the consumer logic of individuals in societies of plenty. And, in the face of the climate crisis and the COVID-19 pandemic, we are called upon to learn to "live with," to get used to the "new normal." What does "living with" mean? What are the rules of this new normality? Here we, transplant recipients, those with a weakened immune system, may be able to help.

I remember the amazement that took hold of me when the first guidelines were published in the beginning of the pandemic and there was general fear of being infected. "Here, suddenly, everyone has a weak immune system. Everyone is like us, the transplant recipients and other patients with weak immune systems," I thought to myself. Vulnerability was becoming the identifying mark of the period, and perhaps the figure representing the cure was that of the chronically ill person, the one with the weak immune system, and the one who was always exposed to injury, danger, and viruses?

In the early days of transplantation medicine, when it was understood that the main challenge to acceptance of an organ was the immune system that attacked every foreign body and that recipients would have to receive a cocktail of medicines that would permanently weaken their immune system, it was posited that recipients would be "bubble people." They would close themselves in their homes and would avoid social and interpersonal contact as much as possible. Life in isolation is better than not living at all, and that is the sole option – they thought in the 1960s and 1970s – for organ recipients, who were endangered by every virus. Every flu or even a simple cold could be fatal for individuals with a suppressed immune system.

Advances in pharmacology, primarily in the more selective manner of suppressing the immune system than in the 1960s and 1980s, refuted the predictions of "bubble people." Today, organ recipients behave much more freely than was predicted, but they are experts, like other chronic patients, at "living with." I can testify about myself as a kidney recipient that I am always extra careful in winter, avoid unnecessary risks, live with a regimen of medicines, and am careful about what I eat and especially about drinking a lot of water. But primarily, I live with the knowledge that the day will come when my body rejects the organs transplanted in me. Nature has its own wisdom that eventually overpowers the cunning of technology. This truth is the challenge underlying transplantation medicine: Finding ways to bypass the self-defense mechanisms of the human immune system is the never-ending scientific front of transplantation medicine. I remember that in the 1990s a new immunosuppressant agent called Prograf was introduced and we were asked whether we were willing to shift from the first-generation medicine (Cyclosporine) to Prograf. I mention this because we are always on the front line of research, ready to participate in the final stage of new technologies. Today, hopes are pinned on gene-editing technologies that will disrupt the mechanism of organ rejection – of organs that perhaps will be taken from animals or printed in 3D bioprinters and will be transplanted in those awaiting an organ. Perhaps, precision medicine will help in engineering organs adapted to the individual's immune system. Either way, we are awaiting the next medical-technological development.

Therefore, when there was concern over the rapid approval of the vaccines against COVID-19, and people were afraid to be vaccinated with a vaccine that had not yet been tried widely over several years, I said to myself, Welcome to the world of those who live on the frontiers of scientific innovation. We know that our lives depend on scientific advances in the field of organ acceptance and are willing to participate in this huge research effort, with all its uncertainty. The COVID-19 pandemic clarified the fact that medical sciences rely on experiments, that medical sciences do not always save lives, that medical technology is not always certain, that science is built on expert critiques, and primarily that it would be naïve to think that medicine is a factory that produces magic bullets that cure everything. I've been an organ recipient since 1986. It's not clear to me how thorough medical knowledge is regarding the long-term effects of the pills I take and the treatments I undergo. Undoubtedly, knowledge about people who underwent transplantation dozens of years ago is very meager, if it exists at all.

The question of the long-term effects arose primarily regarding the vaccines. People refrained from becoming vaccinated because the long-term effects of vaccination are not known. Suddenly, each person adopted what seemed to them as scientific thinking with wording and buzzwords like "long-term effects." What does that really mean? How do you manage your life on the basis of probabilities of a medical event in an unclear range of years? It seems to me that this discourse about the long-term effects of the vaccines is a cover for some fear, the fear of our frailty and vulnerability. The fact is that suddenly everyone became aware that our lives depend on science that we can't really access and that we are required to trust it because the alternative is too difficult and too dangerous.

But we have agency on another level that enables action and a possible way out of the pandemic. Health, the pandemic has taught us, is a social matter. We are dependent on others. In the course of the pandemic, we saw the paradigm of total lockdowns of entire countries. New Zealand closed its skies and was extremely uncompromising in locking down its inhabitants following each verified case of the virus. There were periods in which New Zealand succeeded in escaping from the various variants of COVID-19. The race toward vaccines and medicines also was based on an attitude of vaccine nationalism, and every country sought to set its own unique course for coping with the pandemic. This reflected the Hobbesian logic of "each man for himself" and the rule of the mighty.

But this paradigm failed because the percentage of vaccinated people differed from one place to another and gave rise to new variants that spread quickly. From India, South America, and South Africa – which did not receive the expensive vaccines developed in the West – came the variants that led to global waves of infection and the continuation of the pandemic. International collaboration might have prevented this situation. An understanding of our shared human destiny might have moderated the solipsistic view of "me first, last, and all the time." Vaccines for poor countries would not have come as the result of compassion or justice, but rather from the understanding that the right to overall health includes a commitment to provide access to health resources.

Individuals with a weak immune system include not only transplant recipients or those whose immune system has been weakened by medical treatments. We are the lucky ones, with access to the cutting edge of biomedicine. People with a weakened immune system are also those who have access to the public health system, periodic vaccinations, clean water, and healthful food. The health of those living in the global south or east is perceived by the west as related to a commitment to humanitarian aid, to the volunteerism of individuals or organizations, and to compassion and help through generosity. But the COVID-19 pandemic (like the climate crisis) indicated the direct, shared connection of the health of all. What is required is solidarity, which includes not identification or empathy with the weak but rather deep commitment deriving from the understanding that the dangers and crises are global.

The understanding that "no man is an island entire of itself," is the rationale behind transplantation medicine, not only because of the transplantation of an organ from one body to another but rather because the normative derivative of organ transplantation is solidarity. Without solidarity, there are no organ transplants and we will not succeed in coping with the global crises of the 21st century.

From being a curiosity of heartwarming personal interest stories, the world of transplant recipients has become in recent years a mirror of the distresses and crises befalling us. The "new normal" of life on the verge of danger; the dependence on medical technology, with its positive and negative aspects; the understanding that salvation lies in the willingness of the other to cooperate; and the understanding that our lives are not only a story that we write but rather the outcome of our dependence on the environment and the other – these are the daily experiences of the organ recipient. In this respect, the book before you does recount how organs become available for transplantation, but in this period, its messages seem to be much broader in scope.

The book consists of two styles: an in-depth analysis of the problem of the shortage of organs for transplantation and the political economy that grows out of the problem of the shortage, and shorter biographical sections that tell the stories of my own transplants. Thus far, I have undergone four transplants: in 1986, 1999, 2004, and 2020. Each of the transplantations took place at a different point in the development of transplantation medicine and of the way in which I received the organs. These stories converse with what is described in the academic sections and clarify, from a personal perspective, the political economy of organs for transplantation.

This book is the outcome of the research that was my personal survival project, alongside academic inquiry. The main argument here is that the world of organ transplantation is undergoing a revolution. The growing shortage of organs for transplantation is leading patients and recipient candidates, most of them with kidney disease, to seek solutions on their own. The political economy of organ transplantation is becoming private; it is undergoing privatization. The medical success of organ transplantation has led to tremendous demand for this technology. But, the medical success has not been accompanied by social legitimation: Organ transplantation and organ donation still terrify the public as shady, or at least frightening, medicine. The shortage of organs leads patients to turn to their acquaintances, relatives, and those who admire them, or, alternatively, organ merchants. In all of these cases, the search for an organ for transplantation is a do-it-yourself project. The political economy of organ transplantation indicates the accelerated processes of individualization in the supply of organs for transplantation. These are processes that create a disconnect between the ethos of altruism and solidarity for the common good and the private reality of individual gifts and altruism limited to our relatives. This disconnect is the dominant characteristic of organ transplantation today. But, a full understanding of it requires consideration and understanding of the conditions that move and block the supply of organs for transplantation.

This book describes the structure, conditions, and processes that stir the political economy of organ transplantation. This is an economy based on a tripartite structure consisting of the state, the market, and the family. The individualization of the supply of organs for transplantation is actually the story of the rise of the market and the family as dominant sources of organs for transplantation. This rise, I argue in this book, leads to a major contradiction between the ethos of transplantation and the actual practice of donations from living persons. The moral and ethical discussion regarding the supply of organs for transplantation is shaped by this contradiction.

Acknowledgments

This book is an expansion and reworking of the book *The Plural Me*, which appeared in Hebrew in 2018 (Van Leer Institute Press and Hakibbutz Hameuchad). I would like to thank Prof. Shai Lavi, Van Leer Jerusalem Institute director, and Dr. Tal Kohavi, editor-in-chief of the Van Leer Institute Press, for their willingness to allow me to publish an expanded version of the book in English. The Van Leer Jerusalem Institute is my academic and professional home and I am grateful to my friends at the institute and especially the institute's management for its generosity in helping finance the English translation. More people have accompanied me on my academic journey. Foremost among them is Prof. Yehouda Shenhav, the supervisor of my doctoral thesis, who was always willing to help with a thought or advice. But mainly he served as a source of inspiration. I also wish to thank Prof. Hanna Herzog, who also accompanied me for many years as a devoted supervisor. Prof. Eva Illouz helped me in approaching publishers. Prof. Orly Lobel, a true close friend since we met in junior high, helped and supported me with good advice. Prof. Nadav Davidovitch, Prof. Yael Hashiloni-Dolev, Prof. Dani Filc, Dr. Anat Rosenthal, and Prof. Aviad Raz helped me greatly in my research journey on the paths of the sociology and anthropology of health. This book could not have been written without your reading, comments, and good friendship. Special thanks to Prof. Silke Schicktanz from Goettingen University and Prof. Barbara Prainsack for long conversations on organ donations and transplant medicine.

I am already a senior citizen of the transplantation department at the Rabin Medical Center, and I extend thanks to the dozens of those who have accompanied me on my health obstacle course for decades: the department heads, the nurses, the doctors, transplantation coordinators, administrative staff, and other workers. In particular, I would like to thank Dr. Ruti Rahmimov, Dr. Eviatar Nesher, Prof. Eytan Mor, Dr. Zaki Shapira, Dr. Alexander Yussim, The late Dr. Dani Shmueli, Dr. Shamir Lustig, Rachel Michovich, Dr. Sigal Aizner, Dr. Aviad Greavetz, Dr. Vladimir Tennak, Sigal Cohen, Anat Briger, Dr. Marius Braun, Yael Harif, Tiki Mashraki, Dikla Guri, and Sarit Avidar. The late Rabbi Avraham Heber inspired me greatly with the magnificent living donor project he established and I wish his widow Rachel Heber great success in continuing his life work. The conversations with him, Rachel, and Judy Singer, a kidney donor, taught me a great deal. Many thanks to my close friend Shoham Melamed-Slotman for hours of long conversations and a true friendship.

My beloved family – my parents, David and Ziva; my brothers, Arik and Noam; and my immediate family, my wife Maya and my children, Michael and Nadi – my heart and soul are devoted to you. I can't imagine my life without the support and great love my family gives me.

This book is dedicated to the two organ donors who saved my life. In 2004, I received a kidney under complex circumstances from K., and in 2020, I received a kidney and the liver of an 18-year-old youngster who was killed in a scooter accident. His parents had the inner strength to donate his organs and save me and three other people. It is hard to find the words to describe the sublimity of this noble act. I shall always be grateful.

Jerusalem 1973

When I was born, the only person in my family with a mutation of the PAX2 gene that causes renal dysplasia – a kidney deformation – organ transplants were still a futuristic, experimental, heroically daring technology with limited results. Genetic knowledge was also in its infancy and my genetic mutation was learned of only decades later. History is written backward, so it was difficult to imagine how quickly life was about to change less than one month after I was born in September 1973. I was born in Jerusalem as the younger brother of a two-year-old and the son of young parents in their late twenties. Jerusalem in those days, right before the shock of the Yom Kippur War, was hospitable to young couples like my parents. They were first-generation Israelis, children of immigrants from Europe, who grew up with the young state, which offered them opportunities to acquire professions and establish themselves in its elite. My father, who worked at the treasury, and my mother, who was an occupational therapist, were overjoyed at the birth of their second son.

It was my grandmother, who came to help her daughter, who noticed something was wrong with her grandson. I was 11 days old when they rushed me to the health clinic and from there the family doctor sent us urgently to the hospital. There they learned how poor my condition was. My kidney function indexes showed almost total kidney failure. The doctors were at a loss and gave up hope. They were afraid I would not last the night, and that if I survived, the damage caused by the toxic blood coursing through my body would make me severely handicapped. They advised my parents to leave me in the hospital and say goodbye. My parents remember the doctors telling them: "You are young parents with a healthy child and you can have more children." That advice went over their heads and they insisted on not giving up on me. Renal failure in babies is monitored and treated in the hope of bringing them to functional stability. Dialysis and transplant did not appear to be realistic solutions, and it would be many years until dialysis was given to children and until the first transplant in a child. What were their plans going forward? What did the future hold for me? My parents say they didn't even think of such questions. They focused on the here and now and tried to overcome it.

DOI: 10.4324/9781003288886-1

The "here and now" of September 1973 was replaced by the "here and now" of October 1973 with the outbreak of the Yom Kippur War. My father was called up to the reserves and sent far away from home. My mother is one of the unsung heroes of the war, the women who stayed behind and ran the home front by defending their families and homes. In a state of mounting uncertainty, with fitful telephone communication, my mother held long-distance phone calls with my father and reported to him her visits to the pediatric ward. She recalls the trips in the car with darkened headlights because of the blackout, up and down the steep roads from their Jerusalem neighborhood to Hadassah Hospital, which was outside of the city. The pediatric ward itself was emptied out for the hospitalization of soldiers from the front. Just a handful of babies remained in the ward. When my mother arrived in the morning, full of trepidation, she would check whether the nurses were looking down, avoiding meeting her eyes, as a sign of bad news. It was go crazy or survive, she told me years later. There was nothing but the continuous present of getting through one day after another and hoping for the best.

I managed to survive that night and many more nights thereafter. I was in the hospital for three months and stabilized with kidney function that allowed me to continue living. I, of course, have no real memories from that time, but my parents remember it as a seminal time. My main memory from those years is the bicarbonate solution mixed in hot milk that I drank every morning to balance my blood acidity because of my kidney failure. That was my morning drink, instead of chocolate milk or tea, for years until my first transplant at the age of 13. I celebrated my first birthday in the pediatric ward of the hospital and thereafter paid follow-up visits every few months. My condition continued to be stable and I had an almost normal childhood. My parents' policy was to put my medical condition in parenthesis and let me have a normal childhood. But I was different in many ways. I was short, relatively weak, and had to follow a diet. It was an invisible handicap. It is not easy to explain to a child why he is not allowed to eat certain foods, especially since eating them did not set off an unusual physical reaction. But, when you are a child, you live in a prison of rules that seem arbitrary to you. The mutation I carried also caused a special structure in my left eye, a structure called "morning glory," in which the eye nerve is not fully attached. That structure caused a sort of squint in my left eye and the erroneous assumption of lazy eye. I was even instructed to wear an eye patch for many hours of the day.

That is how I grew up in 1970s Jerusalem. Besides that morning solution, I didn't take any special pills and in any case life was much simpler then, with a routine of school followed by playing at home in the afternoon. Nor did any major medical breakthrough occur at any stage. After the major breakthroughs of heart, pancreas, and liver transplants in the United States in the 1960s, transplant medicine entered a stagnation stage in the 1970s. The progress in the 1960s was mainly in surgical capabilities, but organ acceptance was still very problematic and organ rejection was relatively rapid. Added to that were arguments over the procurement of organs for transplantation. The source of the organs in cases of brain death raised a series of ethical and scientific questions. Can brain death really indicate death? What is the specific place in the brain after whose destruction death can be determined, and is brain death an alibi for organ supply? As we shall see in the following chapters, these questions actually still roil the world of organ transplants, but in those days, along with the difficulty of the rapid rejection of transplanted organs, it brought the transplant industry to a standstill.

The situation in Israel was similar. The first heart transplant took place in the late 1960s, about one year after the first heart transplant in the world. But, already then, ethical issues surrounding the source of the organs came up. Dialysis machines were rare and were still considered an expensive treatment all over the world. For me, and for other children in my condition, the transplant horizon looked very far away and unrealistic. I remember myself, for instance, at the age of 10 or 11, sitting with my grandfather on the balcony of his home in one of the suburbs of Haifa, looking at the backyard garden he loved to cultivate. He stared at a distant point in the air and said to me, as if he were thinking out loud, that if he only could he would give me one of his kidneys. I remember my surprise at hearing that statement. It sounded to me patently preposterous. I don't know if he had even heard of the existence of kidney transplants. Beyond the technological breakthrough of the 1960s, no kidney transplants were performed in Israel at that time. Israeli patients were transplanted at medical centers in Europe and the United States. I think that was the first time that the possibility of a transplant, of a kidney donation, was ever mentioned to me. I attributed the strange idea to my grandfather's gushing sentimentality and actually to the fact that the only practical solution was to continue living in the same way.

The breakthrough that turned transplantation medicine into routine medicine occurred in the early 1980s. It was a real revolution that changed that medicine beyond recognition. The discovery of the attributes of a fungus from which an immunosuppressive substance could be extracted led to the creation of the first generation of immunosuppressant agents called cyclosporine, which delayed the rejection of the transplant for many years. It was a scientific and technological advance that managed to overcome the obstacle of the immune system. Together with an earlier advance of identifying and classifying tissues between donor and recipient, the process of allowing the long-term acceptance of the transplant in the recipient's body was completed. Upon that dramatic advance in transplantation medicine, a legislative effort was made to regulate transplantation medicine that was about to break through beyond the boundaries of experimental medicine. In the first half of the 1980s, for instance, the National Organ Transplant Act (NOTA) was passed in the United States, establishing the organ procurement and transplantation network as a federal network for organ donations on behalf of the US Health Department. NOTA also forbids organ trafficking or any other monetary compensation for transplantation organs.

NOTA was passed as a response to the immunosuppressive revolution. After all, it changed transplantation medicine and actually created a new political economy for that medicine. In the first stage of organ transplants, from the first successes of kidney transplants in the middle 1950s until the revolution of the 1980s, the political economy of transplantation medicine was compatible with experimental medicine. It is a political economy that tries to harness legitimacy and resources in favor of future prospects of a medicine that presents itself as "heroic medicine," one that expands the boundaries of medicine's scientific and technological capacity. It is a political economy that prioritizes support of R&D and ranges from public investment to private investment. Transplantation medicine until the last quarter of the 20th century was largely supported by that kind of political economy.

But, the revolution of the early 1980s heralded in a different political economy. The success in significantly delaying the implant rejection turned transplantation medicine into a resounding success. Whereas until the 1980s, for kidney patients, it was never completely clear whether a transplant was better than dialysis; from that point onward, the question was clearly decided in favor of transplant. Demand for transplants constantly increased, transplantation teams were trained, and organ transplantation centers opened all over the world. Furthermore, over time, as transplantation medicine and post-surgical care improved, organ transplantation became a successful technological solution for a growing number of medical conditions. Above all, the new political economics signaled the main problem of transplantation medicine for the coming years: the problem of the shortage of organs for transplantation.

The increasing demand only highlighted the ethical problems of providing organs for transplantation. The prohibition in NOTA of "compensation" for organs for transplantation sought to prevent organ trafficking, which from the outset of transplantation medicine was a taboo. But, organ trafficking is perhaps only the most extreme of the ethical issues in providing organs. The political economy of organs for transplantation is, at the same time, also a moral economy that created ethical categories such as "donation," "altruism," "gift of life," which sought to place organ supply on a moral plane of giving and donation. Other questions included, for instance, the matter of consent: can consent for organ donation after death be presumed or must active volunteering be expected? And who exactly ought to consent for donation after death be received from? Who does the body of the deceased belong to? And what about the transplantation of kidneys that can be extracted from living people? Is it moral to risk a healthy person in favor of the healing of a sick person? And what are the recipient's ethical duties of protecting the implanted organ? Amazingly, many of those questions still remain open, as living proof that the clear success of a medical technology often involves a twisted labyrinth of ethical and moral questions. In that respect, organ transplantation is one of the first harbingers of a broader revolution in medicine – the revolution of advanced medical technologies, which also includes the development of genetics and genomics in the last decades, the rapid growth of fertility medicine, and the development of the technologies that go with it. In that whole broad spectrum of the development of the medical sciences and advanced technology, questions arise as to the appropriate way to relate to organs, tissues, and cells – ones that move from one body to another through donation, rental, sale, or gift. It is a question not only of proprietary rights and legal definition but of the relationship between one individual and another. That is actually the question that guides me in this book. The political economy of transplantation medicine since the 1980s turned the shortage problem into the main problem of that medicine. It is primarily a social problem which the existing transplant technology has apparently not yet solved. How do you build bridges over the gaping abyss of the shortage and find organs for transplantation?

Of course, none of this concerned me at the time. I was going into the eighth grade in Tel Aviv where we had moved, and besides that single conversation about transplants with my grandfather, I didn't pay much attention to what the future held. I knew my condition, of course, but the farthest I could think ahead was the age of induction to the military. Would I go to the army when I was 18? I wanted to be like everyone else, but who could know? My condition had worsened much earlier. At the age of 12, when my child's body began to signal it wished to develop into an adolescent, my kidneys began to collapse under the strain. I remained skinny, weak, and very short. We still went for checkups every few months at the Jerusalem hospital where I was born and treated, and the indexes pointed to a steady worsening. In 1986, before my bar mitzvah, it was clear things could not go on as they were.

My parents were given a choice between dialysis and transplantation. That was already progress compared to the previous decade, when transplantation was not even on the table. Dialysis could have replaced the kidney's blood-filtering function, but it would not have replaced its hormonal functions, and could have stunted my growth and development. Transplantation appeared to be a better solution, although it was still novel and experimental in the Israeli context. Besides the possibility of traveling to experienced centers abroad, there was also a local option. Beilinson hospital had just opened a new kidney transplantation unit. It included only three physicians and one hospitalization area at the end of the urology department. After consultation and consideration, my parents opted for a transplant at Belinson. The only question that remained was where the kidney would come from. For that matter, where do organs for transplantation come from anyway?

Organ donations from the deceased were extracted at the time under the principle of presumed consent and without a system of transplant coordinators. It was the transplantation doctors themselves who took the organs. It was a problematic situation that led to many clashes (and has since been rectified), and for children, such a source of donation was even more problematic. Actually, the only option that remained was a kidney donation from a living person. My parents were told that as far as rejection of the transplant, the genetic relationship between parents and children guaranteed better acceptance of the kidney. Now, it remained to be decided who would donate, father or mother?

If only the objective indexes could have easily resolved that dilemma. Both of them wanted to do it. Neither of them had many doubts. My father was 42 and my mother was 40 and they were both eligible donors. The compatibility indexes found almost equal genetic compatibility between both of them and myself. My father was slightly more compatible and maybe that is what tipped the scales. My mother says there was also a gender consideration: if birth is the first gift of life, then this was my father's opportunity to give me a second gift of life, a gift of life from him, a sort of "rebirth." There may have also been a preference for a larger kidney that could fulfill the needs of my growing body. My father is tall and strong, and my mother is short and thin. In any case, I was not part of those deliberations and the only thing I knew in the summer of 1986 was that I was getting worse, that I needed to maintain a strict, low-protein diet, and that in the fall, two weeks after my 13th birthday and bar mitzvah ceremony, I was going to undergo a kidney transplant from my father.

I think I was in the first group of children who had kidney transplants in Israel. The surgery was relatively successful. One memory that stayed with me is my father moaning, calling for his mother, and I – at 13 – being amazed that even at 42 people still wanted their mothers. I was in the hospital for two weeks during which a general nursing strike broke out, post-surgical complications left me with a urological problem that would require a long series of surgeries in the future, but the improvement in my condition was rapid and successful. The morning solution I had been drinking since infancy was replaced by cyclosporin – an immunosuppressant agent – which in those days came as a greasy solution that had to be mixed with orange juice to overcome its taste, and a battery of other immunosuppressant pills including steroids, which I still take to this day.

I remember the great admiration my father received after donating the kidney. My grandparents on both sides, who had not been in on the secret, were particularly proud of him. I never talked to my grandfather again about my father's donation and just over a year later he died. Kidney donations from living people were at the time unusual indeed and my father's act drew attention. In the same breath, it was perceived as completely natural, as an almost necessary act. Today, when I am myself the father of children, I understand the almost immediate willingness to help your child in any way. Then, I understood it intuitively and saw transplantation as part of the devotion my parents showed me throughout the years. I didn't feel grateful or that I would stay in perpetual debt to him. Our relationship remained on the spectrum of relationships between parents and adolescent children.

Life after the transplant went back to the track my parents had laid out for me since my childhood: a normal routine of school and a normal social life. The transplant really did improve my life a lot and thanks to it I even managed to reach the height of 165 cm (the greatest achievement of my life…), a little short but tall enough to integrate in society without requiring special explanations. When I was 17 I even met my future wife. I was sure the story was over. Nobody told me that a transplanted kidney is likely to eventually be rejected and that the question of where do organs come from will continue to haunt me. The following chapters suggest a partial answer.

1   Exercising Shortage

The crisis of transplantation medicine

Organ shortage is the hallmark of transplantation medicine. It is the main obstacle facing medicine, and it overshadows the surgical successes and scientific victories that make it possible to transplant an organ from one body into another. In the shadow of the organ shortage, transplantation medicine seems like an empty technology, an instrument waiting to be used. The gap between the great promise inherent in transplantation medicine and the ongoing crisis rooted in shortage may be one of the major ironies of modern medicine. We might say that it is shortage that is the generator of the biggest drama in the social history of transplantation medicine, and it is that shortage that is at the basis of the analysis in this work.

At the end of the 20th century, transplantation technology became a sort of wonder cure for a growing number of medical conditions, and today it redeems patients in advanced stages of heart failure, renal failure, liver diseases, and many other chronic conditions. The more transplantation medicine expands and thrives, the greater the demand for organs and the deeper the scarcity. The rise in the incidence of growing chronic diseases throughout the world exacerbates further the shortage (Geneau, Stuckler, Stachenko et al. 2010). The increasing incidence of diseases such as diabetes and hypertension in developing countries such as India and Pakistan, along with the development of transplantation medicine in those countries as well, has turned the shortage of organs for transplantation into a global problem (Rizvi, Naqvi, Zafar et al. 2003). The success of transplantation medicine, on the one hand, and the shortage of organs for transplantation, on the other hand, create the tension that drives the political economy of transplantation organs. The contours of this political economy will be unfolded in the following chapters, but at this stage, exploring the dynamics of organ shortage, its origins, and the ethics it generates is necessary for a full comprehension of what is organ economy.

Figure 1.1 shows simply and straightforwardly the rise in the transplant waiting list in the United States from 1988 to 2019. The figure shows that the number of people waiting for organ transplants rose sharply over the years, whereas the number of actual donors and the number of transplants performed rose only

DOI: 10.4324/9781003288886-2

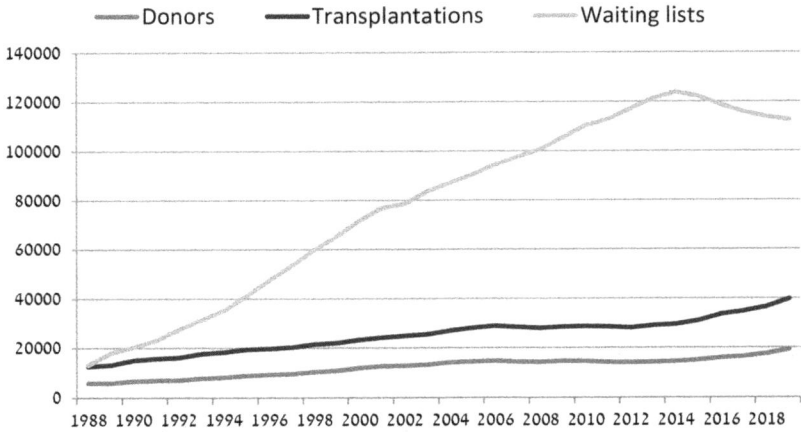

Figure 1.1 Waiting list, donations, and transplantations in the United States 1988–2019
Source: http://optn.transplant.hrsa.gov

moderately: during those years, the waiting list grew more than eightfold, but the number of transplants rose by a factor of only 3.14. At the end of 2019, the number of people waiting for transplants in the United States alone was more than 112,000, but only a little less than 40,000 transplants were performed that year, a ratio of about 1:3. We must remember that getting on the waiting list depends on the inability to rehabilitate the defective organ. In the case of a kidney, for instance, only dialysis patients get on the list. Therefore, people waiting for transplants are in mortal danger, or at the very least at risk of failure of body systems, and their quality of life is poor.

The limited supply of organs for transplantation seems surprising, since most of the organs are harvested from cadavers, and one could have thought that an economy based on organs from deceased people – even if it requires a special definition of death – would have an almost unlimited supply. Figure 1.2 shows how far that perception is from reality. In 1988, the ratio between people waiting for transplants and actual transplants in the United States was 0.96 so that almost every person on the waiting list got a transplant; in 2000, the ratio was 0.32 so that only 32 transplants were performed for every 100 people waiting; and in 2019, the ratio was 0.35, after a low of 0.24 in 2014. The shortage deepened in particular in the 1990s. It was in that decade that transplantation medicine established itself as a routine practice with very high success rates. Transplant surgery led to a significant improvement in the quality of life of patients with terminal chronic diseases and to a considerable extension of their life expectancy. Indeed, since the first decade of the 21st century, the worsening of the shortage problem slowed down a little, and in the second decade, a slight change in the trajectory can be seen. But, these changes are negligible in relation to the demand for organs

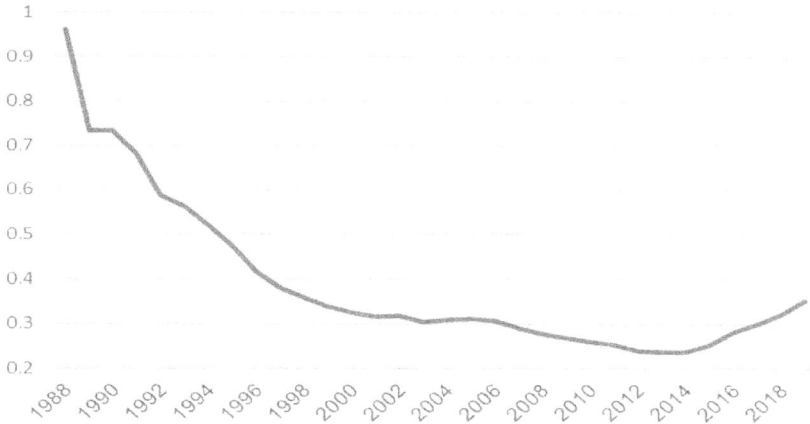

Figure 1.2 The ratio between people on waiting lists and actual transplants in the United States 1988–2019
Source: http://optn.transplant.hrsa.gov

for transplantation, and organ shortage remains the hallmark of transplantation medicine in this century as well.

The demand for organs is ever increasing and the gap remains insurmountable. The scarcity of organ donations does not stem from donor scarcity alone, but also from some structural constraints. Certain organs, especially the heart and pancreas, can only be harvested from the bodies of the deceased. "Some must die," wrote ethicist Stuart Youngner in a well-put summary of the main ethical dilemma of transplantation medicine (Youngner 2003). The fact that saving the life of one person involves the death of another raises moral and ethical questions that require extensive consideration. These questions are related mainly to the fact that the optimal organ donation occurs in the case of brain death. I will discuss the definition of brain death, its relationship to transplantation medicine, and the ethical issues that arise from it later on. But for the matter at hand, I will say that the dependence on the definition of brain death limits as the main source for organs, limits the supply of donations.

A study that examined the number of cases of brain death in the United States estimated that every year between 10,500 and 13,000 such cases are diagnosed (Sheehy, Suzanne, Conrad et al. 2003). A more recent study estimated that between 1% and 2% of all death in the United States are brain death (Spinello 2015). In 2018, donations after brain death increased to 8,591, from 8,403 in 2017 in the United States; this number has been increasing since 2012.[1] The progress in the early diagnosis of symptoms of stroke, and the drop in the number of fatal traffic accidents thanks to the safety features required from vehicle manufacturers, reduced the supply of transplantation organs even further and worsened the shortage, and this was evident in the late 1980s (Annas 1988). The decline in cases of brain death led to attempts to expand the potential pool of donors to include cardiac death and not only brain death. Furthermore, given the progress in the development of immunosuppressant drugs and post-transplant therapy, harvesting organs from cadavers that were previously not considered good candidates for donation became possible (Keizer, De Fijter, Haase-Kromwijk et al. 2005, Abt, Desai, Crawford et al. 2004). But even after the possibilities of post-mortem organ donation were expanded, the shortage remained intact.

Again, the patients waiting for transplants have already reached the terminal phase of their diseases. Given the limited supply, merely getting on the waiting list is limited to the most serious cases. Many patients have not yet reached that stage, but they are precisely the ones who might benefit more from a transplant and enjoy an improvement in their quality of life for a longer time than those who are already sicker. If we counted those patients as well in the number of people waiting, the ratio between patients waiting for transplants and actual transplants in the United States would be even higher. Therefore, the organ shortage is much deeper and more extensive than the statistics show. According to the US National Kidney Foundation, in the United States alone, there are nearly 660,000 patients treated for terminal kidney diseases.[2] The vast majority of them have not yet been put on the organ transplant waiting list. According to accepted medical ethics, the correct way to measure the shortage is based on the number of the most urgent patients. But, it is precisely the broader extent of the shortage that shapes the patterns of the organ economy. What, then, is the sociological and political significance of that economy?

Every economy is to some extent an economy of shortage. Shortage is the organizing principle of any economy, and the regulation of a shortage is the essence of an economic activity. The ratio between supply and demand sets off a series of exchange patterns that form what we understand as "economy." This is the essence of economies everywhere from exchange to market economies. But unlike other economies, in which the ratio between supply and demand is flexible and changeable, shortage in the organ economy is rigid, constant, and worsening (Cook and Krawiec 2014). Moreover, in the case of the organ economy, it cannot be simply described as merely a question of supply and demand. Talking about human organs as if they were objects of economic analysis seems inappropriate. Commodities and exchangeable objects are not charged with meanings of dignity as the human body does, and this alone renders the jargon of economics unfit for discussing the exchange of organs between the person in the process of transplantations (Dickenson 2017, Radin 1987). Applying an economic theory requires an adaptation. Concepts like "shortage," "supply," and "demand" are applied by economists to any sort of markets as if the market's substance of exchange serves the conceptual framing. It does work for many markets in highly consumerist as ours but cannot be applied directly and without adjustments to the problem of organs for transplants.

The "supply"/"demand" categorization is criticized from yet another perspective. Organ shortage – the critic goes – is not a problem of low supply to high demand. This is perhaps the tip of the iceberg, a mystification of much deeper social problem. The lack of organs for transplantations is the result of the cultural and social inacceptability of organ transplantation. Organ scarcity is seen as a vote of no confidence in a medical western technology that overstepped sacred taboos such as the definition of life and death, the anthropomorphism axiom, and bodily integrity. In Chapter 2, I explore more extensively this line of criticism.

The two opposing perspectives on transplantation medicine, the one who applies theories and tools from economics to explore and solve the shortage problem, and the critical, who sees transplantation as a transgressive medical technology, draw the main two dominant discourses on transplantation in the social sciences. It seems that any discussion on transplantation medicine cannot proceed without choosing between the two. Adapting the economic perspective leads the researcher into suggesting normative and practical ways of overcoming the shortage problem. From the critical perspective, transplantation medicine calls for a more fundamental exploration into the relations between advanced medical technologies and society. The first approach views the shortage as a problem of procuring and allocating healthcare resources, whereas the second approach views it as an expression of the impact of modern medicine and technology on society.

Every discussion of transplantation medicine requires, declaratively or implicitly, a normative choice about the position of that medicine in the social fabric. The fact that transplantation medicine requires the transfer of an organ from one person to another puts it on a social footing and renders it impossible to avoid making a normative choice.

As a subject in this dark kingdom of shortage, the practical orientation of the economic and institutional approach is more appealing. It frames the suffering of waiting for a donation, as an organizational problem or an issue that can be solved with the right policy. As if the solution waits there. But as a sociologist, I know that there is much more into the problem of organ shortage. There is a certain truth in arguing that this technology is not just like any other medical treatment. It involves the removal of an organ from another person. Such medicine cannot exist without the public's cooperation in the most literal sense: it is the public that provides the organs for transplantation and the same public that creates the shortage. It is useless without the public's compliance and acceptance. Already at the very beginning of transplantation medicine, in the 1950s and 1960s, it was evident that the issue of organ supply is the main challenge for that medicine's development. Many believed, and some still do, that the challenge could be overcome by technological, normative, and legal adjustments, changes, and innovations. But actually, the shortage gave rise to a new ethical order. That ethical order developed simultaneously with the development of transplantation medicine. I need a deeper understanding of how the ethics of transplantations develops in order to find myself the right footing both as an organ recipient and as a social scientist. This is my task in this chapter where I will demonstrate how the organ shortage emerged as a specific case of healthcare resource distribution and how it came to embody the dilemmas of the medicine–society relationship in the age of advanced medical technologies.

Exercising shortage: the creation of a new ethical order

The most significant breakthroughs in transplantation medicine occurred in the 1950s and 1960s. In 1954, a successful kidney transplant was performed between twins. In 1967, the first liver transplant was performed in the United States. At the same year the first heart was transplanted by a team headed by Christiane Bernard in Cape Town, South Africa. These medical successes, as often happen with pioneering technologies, lacked the ethical envelope to justify both the investment and the result. Kidney transplants, which were the vanguard of transplantation medicine, developed a few years after the invention of the dialysis machine ("the artificial kidney"), which provided a parallel solution to the problem of kidney failure. The parallel development of the two technologies allows an examination of the formation of the ethical framework for addressing the question of shortage in an era of advanced medical technologies.

In the early 1960s, both kidney transplants and dialysis machines had limited success in saving the lives of terminal kidney disease patients, and both contended with normative uncertainty. One of the best examples is the question of patient selection for the artificial kidney treatment. This was one of the first questions that defined medical ethics as a field that is also concerned with the distribution of health resources in conditions of shortage. In 1962, the first dialysis clinic in the world opened in Seattle, but the small experimental clinic could not treat the numerous terminal kidney patients. Belding H. Scribner, the clinic director, decided to solve the problem of patient selection in worsening conditions of shortage by forming a committee. The committee comprised two physicians and five public representatives: a clergyman, a lawyer, a housewife, a union leader, and a government official. The committee was modeled after the US jury system, where a decision is made after an open normative discussion in light of two medical experts' recommendations. The considerations for the selection of the first five patients to receive the new technology were published in Life Magazine in November 1962 (Alexander 1962). Besides a series of medical criteria, the considerations were age, family status, education, income, mental stability, occupation, previous professional attainments and estimated future attainments, and personal reputation, determined by recommendations of the candidates' associates (Alexander 1962). In addition, the committee decided that only the residents of Washington state were entitled to dialysis treatments because the technology was funded by the taxes they paid. It was also decided that the dialysis treatment would not be approved for people older than 45, nor for children because according to the committee members they lacked the necessary resilience for such a difficult and intensive treatment (Blagg 1999, Darrah 1987). These criteria were known as the "social worth" component of selecting candidates for the medical treatment (Jonsen 1998).

A report about the committee, under the heading "they decide who lives and who dies," stirred an outcry. The report quoted committee members admitting that their decisions were largely arbitrary and that they actually had no clear guidelines on how to decide who was entitled to treatment and who was not. In response, a call went out to philosophers, jurists, theologians, and physicians to establish more solid criteria of entitlement to treatment with the artificial kidney in particular, and rare healthcare resources in general, on the basis of professional knowledge. The main outcry was against the social worth component: David Sanders and Jesse Dukeminier viewed the committee's criteria as a reflection of middle-class morality; others tried to formulate more abstract principles for patient selection (Sanders and Dukeminier 1967, Childress 1970, Rescher 1969, Schreiner 1966). Albert Jonsen, one of the most important historians of bioethics, views the response to the Seattle committee as the birth of bioethics, because it created a new field of discourse combining religious, philosophical, and legal principles to form a system of rules that could be applied to other cases concerning the distribution of healthcare resources (Blagg 1999, Darrah 1987). Renée Fox and Judith Swazey, medical anthropologists who conducted historic research of the early days of dialysis, also assert that the Seattle committee was the cradle of Western bioethics (Fox and Swazey 1974).

Technological developments during the 1960s that improved the artificial kidney made the treatment less arduous for patients and made it possible to expand the pool of patients. Nonetheless, the question of entitlement or deservingness to treatment in a reality of increasing demand remained a challenge for healthcare policymakers. In 1964, at the Mayo Clinic in Washington, DC, the following criteria for entitlement to dialysis treatment were set forth: adult candidate aged 18–55, suffering from terminal kidney disease without complications or other illnesses, emotionally stable and able to cooperate, someone who can offer a candidate for a kidney donation. These criteria also included the element of social worth, and the impact of the emerging ethical discourse on them was still weak. But, the last condition – the ability to propose a candidate for kidney donation – is interesting. It indicates that even then dialysis treatment was a preparation stage before kidney transplantation and that it developed simultaneously with transplantation medicine. The artificial kidney (dialysis) remained a solution for terminal kidney patients, but the kidney transplant offered a much broader horizon, because it attested to the great potential in the development of organ transplant technology, in general.

The new moral economy that was developed surrounding the use of innovative technologies, at that time, was soon to become what is known today as bioethics. In this emerging field, the question of who gets to be treated with these new technologies touches on the issues of redistribution and justice in rare health resources distribution. Transplantation medicine added another layer to this question: it is not only advanced medical technologies that are rare, so are human organs for transplantation. Even though the use of cadavers was an inseparable part of the development of modern medicine as scientific medicine, the use of organs for the experimental transplantation medicine still required a complicated ethical maneuvering.

During those very same years, in 1964, the Helsinki declaration on human experimentation was being articulated, based on the 1947 Nuremberg code. The Declaration of Helsinki, and the changes that were eventually introduced to it, did not directly address the distribution of resources under conditions of shortage, but created the bioethical climate in which that question was expected to be clarified.

The first successes of transplant medicine, their media coverage, and appeal as the apex of modern medicine expanded widely the horizon of transplantation medicine during the 1960s. It also changed the focus of the ethical discussion – from the question of allocation of dialysis treatments to the question of the supply of transplantable organs. The nature of the discussion itself did not change, and stayed on the plane of the allocation of healthcare resources in conditions of shortage. However, the use of tools from the area of the ethics of shortage in order to formulate an ethics concerning the supply of human organs for transplant seemed inappropriate and called for adaptations. First, the fact that the organs that were used in the experimental transplantations of the 1960s came from living persons. This, allegedly, solved the ethical problem of allocation, but already then concerns about coercion and exploitation in living organ "donations" from disempowered groups were raised. Thomas Starzl, the pioneering surgeon of liver transplants and the leader of the transplantation medicine community at its inception, wrote in his memoir:

> Even though I was one of the first to use living kidney donors, and no person who donated a kidney through me ever died, the discussion of the risk that donors might be exploited or coerced agitated me. Over the years, the idea of donation from a living person has seemed to me less and less appropriate [...] Since 1971 I have completely avoided transplanting organs donated by living people.
> (Starzl 1992:147)

Besides the risk of exploitation and coercion, kidney donations from living people created a severe ethical problem. Removing a kidney from a healthy individual violates the first rule of medical ethics from the time of ancient Greece: "First, do no harm." Nor is it consistent with the Kantian imperative not to treat human beings as means toward an end. Therefore, the use of organs taken from dead bodies had several advantages: it allowed harvesting additional organs for transplantation (the heart, liver, and pancreas, all at the same time), and it did not violate the ethical prohibition against causing harm to a healthy person, and it avoided the risk of exploitation and coercion inherent in living donations. It seemed as if taking organs from cadavers could solve the shortage problem. At that time, the question of informed consent had not yet been discussed in the context of postmortem organ harvesting. Consent to post-mortem organ removal for therapeutic objectives was presumed at best and usually irrelevant. According to this approach, taking organs from bodies did not violate the ethical guidelines of medical practice during the 1960s and 1970s. However, it did raise another problem: how can you harvest a beating heart for transplantation? After all, if the heart is still beating, the body is not dead. The question of the organ source remained without a clear answer, and ethical exercises and new ethical guidelines were needed in order to answer it and thereby resolve the shortage problem.

Exercising death: the dead donor rule

The successful experiments with heart, liver, and pancreas transplantations during the 1960s highlighted the problem of the source of the organs. These organs are taken only from dead bodies (only in the late 1980s did the use of liver donations from living donors begin), but for them to be worthy of transplantation, the cessation of blood flow into them (ischemia) has to be as brief as possible. The longer the blood flow stops, the greater the damage to the organ until it becomes unsuitable for transplantation. Therefore, the best source of organs for transplantation is the paradoxical state of the still-living body of a dead person. Such cases began to appear in the second half of the 20th century, with the invention of ventilators and defibrillators. In fact, a new state of being (or not being) was created: patients whose hearts continued to beat, but whose brains were destroyed beyond repair. The existence of these people, who received names such as the "living dead," "living cadavers," or the "limbo people," led to a reexamination of the traditional definitions of death and changed the course of the history of organ transplantation.

Medical protocols had always established death based on the absence of cardiac function or nonbreathing. The paradigmatic shift toward a neurological definition of death, which was eventually called "brain death," occurred in the second half of the 20th century, with the publication of the conclusions of an expert committee from Harvard Medical School on "irreversible coma" in 1968 (Beecher 1968). The term "brain death" appeared in the subtitle of the report. During that time, the concepts and nomenclature in that field were in the process of crystallizing into coherent terms, and the term "brain death" was often replaced with the term "coma depassé." Both terms refer to the same condition that required clarification and definition. Historians who traced the committee's work connect the definition of brain death with transplantation medicine (Belkin 2003, Pernick 1999, Giacomini 1997). It is commonly argued that the definition of brain death, which made it possible to harvest organs for transplantation, served the interests of the burgeoning transplantation medicine.

In its recommendations, the Harvard committee presented three conditions for establishing brain death: inability to breathe independently, nonactivity of the reflexes, and absence of electrical brain activity.[3] The purpose of these recommendations was to clarify the obscure status of patients who were "beyond coma" and define them as dead. In 1981, the President's Commission for the Study of Ethical Problems in Medicine and Biomedical and Behavioral Research endorsed the concept of brain death and a pivotal philosophical defense was articulated by the work of James Bernat, Charles Culver, and Bernard Gert (Bernat, Culver and Gert 1981). But not only did these definitions not simplify the complicated situation, to the contrary, they gave rise to new disputes and ambiguities that sowed confusion on the question of death, within and outside the medical community (Youngner, Arnold and Schapiro 2002).[4] One dispute concerned the anatomical aspect of the definition of death: what happens when only part of the brain is irreversibly gone? Or to put it differently, which brain functions are vital to life, and the cessation of which allows declaration of death, and which are not? (Bernat 1992). Another dispute concerned the authority to define death, and was articulated most clearly by Robert Veach, as soon as the committee finished its work. Veach warned against the spillage of the professional debate over the anatomical location of death into overly sweeping definitions of life and death that would be mechanically formulated by physicians. The question of the end of life is primarily a philosophical and ethical question, and the attempt to define the physical area of the brain whose functioning indicates life was perceived as a reduction of the concept of life to a mechanical definition, he argued.[5] Actually, Veach sought to turn bioethics into the organizing axis of the definition of brain death.

The question of the definition of brain death was one of the first areas in which a clear separation was created between bioethics and medical ethics. Bioethics added considerations of a different order to the professional and technological definitions. It sought to disrupt the link between the definition of brain death and organ transplants, through "the dead donor rule." Gary Belkin argues that disruption is one of the main factors in the development of bioethics. He suggests that, in fact, the definition of brain death arose from a large number of clinical and technological factors and that the justifications for that definition derived from differing ethical, professional, and theological philosophies (Belkin 2014, 2003).

A broad discussion of the definition of death in relation to organ transplants had taken place two years before the Harvard committee, at the 1966 Ciba Symposium. At that time, as transplantation medicine was expanding, legal and ethical questions about the procurement methods and policies of transplantation organs had arisen. In a retrospective summary 50 years after the symposium, Ross and Thistlethwaite claimed that the main question that interested the participants was the definition of death (Ross and Thistlethwaite 2016). Therefore, it is evident that two years before the formal definition of brain death, and more than 50 years later, the connection between care for the dying and organ transplants was obvious, and it remained one of the main ethical problems in conflating a scientific definition of death and an ethical problem of organ shortage. As we shall see later on in the following chapters and specifically in examining the Israeli case, this juxtaposition never disappeared, or in the words of ethicist Alexander Capron, "brain death – well settled yet still unresolved" (Capron 2001).

Following some failures in heart transplants during the early 1970s, and the inability to overcome transplant rejection by the immune system, transplantation medicine was caught in a stalemate. The achievements of the 1960s were dulled by the short lifespan and poor quality of life of the transplantees, as a result of the numerous and complicated treatments geared at weakening their immune systems. Besides the disputes over the definition of brain death, transplantation medicine in the 1970s could not shake its characterization as experimental medicine. Only in the late 1970s and early 1980s did it manage to overcome the obstacle of the immune system's resistance and almost overnight became a widespread and routine medicine. At this stage, transplantation medicine needed to bolster its legitimacy, and the "dead donor rule" served this purpose. The purpose of the rule was to gain public trust in transplantation medicine and encourage postmortem organ donation, and it was rewritten as the main precept of the ethics of transplantation medicine (Robertson 1999).

The dead donor rule is to a large extent the first precept in the supply of organs from dead bodies. As its name indicates, it asserts that the donor must be dead. It would seem to be a simple and trivial rule, but it is far from it and its implementation runs up against numerous difficulties, especially because of the dispute over the definition of death (Truog and Miller 2008, Truog and Robinson 2003). Is brain death defined as death? Who is authorized to decide that? To what extent the medical definition of brain death enjoys social legitimization? How to bolster trust in a new definition of death and ensure that it will not be conceived as an alibi for organ retrieval for transplants? These are the questions not only at the basis of worldwide legislation and regulation concerning brain death but also at the basis of the ethical principle that separates between the definition of death and harvesting organs from the dead. The dead donor rule requires a systematic procedure before determining death for the purpose of organ donation; organs cannot be harvested for transplant before reaching consensus on the death itself. In practical terms, the dead donor rule distinguishes between the intensive care unit personnel who determine the death, and the transplantation unit personnel. The latter are not supposed to even know about critical casualties arriving at the ICU until their death is called. When there is disagreement over the question whether a particular patient is in the condition of brain death, the dead donor rule prevents organ donation. To a large extent, the purpose of the rule is to prevent the intrusion of ulterior motives, including the possibility of organ donation, into the process of determining death. From another, perhaps complementary perspective, the dead donor rule can be considered a guarantee of the credibility of the medical establishment toward the public concerning determining death, thereby increasing the number of donors. This achieves a twofold goal: complete consent over the fact of death and encouragement of organ donation as a result of that consent. But as we shall see below, complete consent over the fact of death, especially in cases of brain death, is, sometimes, very difficult to reach.

The dead donor rule declaratively refrains from addressing the shortage problem, and its main effect is to obfuscate the dispute over brain death and conceal it with an ethical rule. It is an ethical machination to deal with the shortage, because it is supposed to alleviate the fear of organs being harvested for transplant before death. The unequivocal wording of the rule and its presentation as the central precept in the ethics of organ donations are meant to play down the argument over the definition of brain death in order to encourage organ donation. In fact, the rule problematizes the concept of death rather than its allegedly simple wording: if the body is dead, what good would it be to harvest its organs for transplant? After all, for the transplant to have high prospects of success, the vitality of the transplanted organ must be maintained by a blood flow. Actually, the rule covers up the fact that in the case of brain death the body is still alive (even if it is kept alive artificially), while the medical protocol establishes death.

One of the ways to overcome the internal contradiction of the dead donor rule is to identify the meeting point between the social–cultural definitions of death and its medical definitions. Cardiac death is a very good example of that meeting point. In the case of cardiac death, the dead donor rule does not involve a contradiction because now the heart is no longer beating, and the transplant takes place immediately. Ethicists, physicians, and policymakers, therefore, wish to expand the pool of potential donors by approaching families whose relatives died cardiac death (Steinbrook 2007). Another, less successful example of the meeting point between the social–cultural definitions of death and its medical definitions is respiratory-brain death, as it has been defined in Israel. This subject will be discussed extensively in Chapter 6.

Exercising consent: what are the wishes of the dead?

In 2017, the French policy of procuring organs for transplantation was reversed. From a policy of explicit consent for donation, through a donor card and a database of citizens willing to donate their organs after their death, France changed to a policy in which consent to donate is the default presumption. Since January 1, 2017, every French citizen is considered to be willing to donate their organs after death, unless having expressed objection to doing so during their life. Those who oppose donation must declare so and be registered in the registrar of people who refuse to donate their organs after death. A similar policy, of presumed consent, has been in force for years in Spain, Austria, and other countries throughout the world. Across the channel, the United Kingdom in 2008 rejected the transition to a policy of presumed consent and retained the policy of informed consent, which requires active consent to organ donation. In 2015, Wales adopted a soft informed consent policy, where there is still a database of people who expressed active consent to donate organs, along with a database of people who refuse to donate. In 2019, the Scottish organ donation bill has been changed to an opt-out system, and a year later, in 2020, The English parliament has joined in and also authorized a transition to presumed consent policy, rendering the whole British Island a presumed consent territory. Thus when a resident of Wales, England, or Scotland is not registered in either database, the presumption is that they consent to organ donation, unless the family vetoes the donation. This all follows EU recommendations, due to concern over the lack of organ donations and the growing shortage of organs for transplant. Indeed, as expected, studies show that a policy of presumed consent yields more organs for donation than a policy of informed consent (Luke, Wesley, Tapper et al. 2019; Usman, Afif, Ahmed-Zayn et al. 2019, Abadie and Gay 2006).

Indecision and policy reversals concerning the consent question and the wishes of the deceased have accompanied organ procurement policy from its inception, and are seen all over the world (Arshad, Anderson and Sharif 2019). They are unique to transplantation medicine and not typical of other areas of healthcare policy. It is the only therapeutical medicine that debates the question of the wishes of the deceased and demonstrates such a volatile and ambivalent policy regarding these wishes. This is, of course, directly related to the shortage problem and to ways to solve it, or at least to reduce its severity. Debating donation consent accompanies transplantation medicine from its inception in the 1960s. An extensive discussion of the legal and ethical issues involved in the procurement of transplantation organs already took place at the Ciba Symposium in 1966. Besides the definition of death, the symposium also discussed the issue of free will and consent to donation concerning living donors, especially given the fear of exploitation of vulnerable groups such as children and prisoners. It is interesting to note that the symposium participants viewed organ donations from living donors as a short-term source. They were sure that the main source of organs would be dead bodies, among other things because of the complex ethical issues surrounding living donations. Joseph Murray who was the first to perform a successful kidney transplant from a living donor in 1954 – the recipient's identical twin – tended to rule out donations from living donors because of the mutilation it causes the donor. He was quoted as saying: "All clinicians working with kidney transplantation should strive for better [deceased donor] organ procurement so that the day will come when even identical twins will not require a living donor" (Ross and Thistlethwaite 2016:1193). Unlike the prophecy about lack of consent on the definition of brain death, on this matter, as we shall see below, Murray's prediction was far from coming true.

The discussion of the question of consent to organ donation from the dead developed as a complement to the dead donor rule, and both questions are intertwined in a tight knot it is hard to tease apart. The consent applies to the act of organ donation but not to determining the moment of death. Is a person who expresses positive consent to donate their organs after their death aware of the dispute over determining brain death? And can a person's consent to donate their organs after death be presumed given there is no consensus on the determination of death? Does consent, informed or presumed, take into account the scientific-clinical complexity of determining brain death? It would appear that the question of defining death is a clinical issue whereas the question of consent is an ethical issue. But as we shall see below, when it comes to organ donation from the dead, the ethical and scientific are intertwined, especially given the doubts over the definition of brain death.

The 1966 international symposium can be seen as the starting point of the ethical discussion on how to harvest organs for transplantation. It was the first conference that discussed, by definition, the legal and ethical aspects of organ transplantation and was attended primarily by physicians from all over the world. It discussed the questions of consent and free will extensively. It was two years after the Helsinki conference that made autonomy – through the concept of informed consent – into a binding ethical principle. The concept of informed consent transformed from a medical norm, as it had developed since the second half of the 19th century in the United States, into a legal criterion (Beauchamp 2004). In the direct sense, the question of consent was associated in the early 1960s with the patient's autonomy to make medical decisions. Until then, since it was merely a norm concerning the appropriate relationship between physician and patient, consent was not a legal requirement, and even when the patient was asked to give their consent, they were not given all of the necessary information in order to make an informed decision. Decisions on treatment remained the purview of the scientists and the patient had no say. For example, patients did not receive information about experiments in which they took part, and disempowered populations participated in medical experiments without their consent. But even after establishing the medical ethics concerning the patient's consent to treatment or participation in experiments – in the Declaration of Helsinki and its amendments – the ethical duty was not always fulfilled when it came to disempowered communities or in non-Western countries. One infamous example is the Tuskegee syphilis experiments, in which poor black patients participated in experiments that tested the "natural" course of the disease, without telling them there was a cure. The patients' consent to participate in the experiment was obtained in exchange for hot meals, free medical care (but not for syphilis), and the commitment to pay for their burial (Gray 1998). The Tuskegee experiments, which began in 1932, drew attention in the mid-1960s, with the emergence of the informed consent norm, and were completely stopped in 1972 after causing a scandal. Experiments of that sort are also cornerstones in the crystallization of informed consent into a legal obligation.

Informed consent became a central plank of medical ethics after a series of committees and decisions, the most famous of which are the 1964 Declaration of Helsinki on human experiments and the Belmont Committee, which was established following the Tuskegee scandal. The combination of those committees and decisions gave rise to the concept of "patient's rights" as a central legal criterion in physician–patient relations. The Declaration of Helsinki, which was based on a code written following the Nuremberg trials, introduced the issue of informed consent in the context of participating in medical research. Its assumption was that making a conscious and informed decision about medical care is directly related to human dignity, and failing to provide the opportunity to make a decision of that nature exceeds the question of medical ethics to the point of violating human dignity. The informed consent model developed mainly out of a series of US rulings on the duty to inform. A review of those rulings shows that the patronizing model, that sees no cause for providing the patient with information, let alone for the patient's discretion, changed gradually to the autonomous model, where formal consent is insufficient and informed consent is required. This means at the very least giving both sides equal weight in making the decision about the desirable treatment, or even giving extra weight to the patient in decisions about treatment and transferring responsibility for the decision to the patient.

The appearance of informed consent as a legal concept led to autonomy taking hold as the paradigm of medical ethics and physician–patient relations. The bioethics that has developed since then has reflected the liberal values that emphasize individual freedom, pluralism, rationality, and free will and thought. The infiltration of these principles into the field of medicine was initially met with suspicion and hostility (Gray 1998), but ultimately, they took hold and became the foundation of the physician–patient relationship, especially in the West. In the 1970s and 1980s, with the appearance of advanced medical technologies such as IVF, developments in genetic science and its applications, and the advent of essential questions about brain death, ventilators, dialysis, and more, a deepening gap emerged between medical ethics, which was concerned with the ethical aspects of the medical profession, and bioethics, which was concerned with the principled dilemmas arising from the practice of medicine. The new medical technologies created a reality in which medical intervention could change accepted perceptions of the course of life, its beginning, and its end. Bioethics contended with the new technologies by translating them into philosophical questions and legal issues, thereby shaping the salient features of the Western bioethical discourse: this included emphasizing liberal principles, creating an abstract ideological context, and a methodology drawn from analytical philosophy. At the basis of liberal bioethics is the principal paradigm that establishes the appropriate medical procedure in a range of situations based on normative basic principles: respect for autonomy, beneficence, nonmaleficence, and justice (Beauchamp and Childress 2001). Informed consent is the legal manifestation of the principle of autonomy. Conceptual and political tension may arise between those principles, but they seem crystallized mainly thanks to the theoretical work that organizes their discussion.

Liberal bioethics draws a straight line between informed consent and participation in medical research, as it has developed since the Declaration of Helsinki, and between informed consent and medical care as a basic principle of the physician–patient relationship. There are supposedly two models of informed consent that developed from two different historical sources, one concerning medical research and the other medical treatment. In fact, the two sources have merged into one model of informed consent as it is currently known in Western bioethics. Transplantation medicine is a perfect example of that historical process. After all, until the 1980s, before the breakthrough in immunosuppressant therapy, organ transplantation was considered experimental medicine, and consent to an organ transplant equaled consent to participate in medical research. Since the 1980s, transplantation medicine has been perceived as routine medicine and consent to a transplant is tantamount to consent to treatment.

A look at the development of the principles of bioethics in the 1960s and 1970s in the United States, especially at Georgetown University, the nearby Kennedy Center of Ethics, and the Hastings Center, reveals a clear picture at the center of which is an individual person with free thought and discretion (Beauchamp and Childress 2001). Among the principles of liberal bioethics, or the "Georgetown principles," the principle of autonomy occupies a pride of place that sometimes overshadows other principles such as justice or avoiding harm. The principle of autonomy allows the patient to decide on a different course of treatment than the physician suggested and also justifies private, unequal medicine according to the market principle, based on the patients' free will.

It is important to trace the history of the concept of informed consent because transplantation medicine challenges that principle for several reasons. First, as we saw above, the history of transplantation medicine is a perfect example of the blurring of the difference between informed consent to medical research and informed consent to medical treatment. Such blurring is typical to many advanced medical technologies at their inception. Until recently, and in many places even today, postmortem organ donation is tantamount to donating one's body to science. It is a relic of the concept of organ transplantation as experimental medicine, and of consent to donation as consent to participation in research.

Second, informed consent to donate organs after death raises the philosophical question about the wishes of the deceased. What is the meaning of consenting to an act after death? How is the wish of the deceased determined? A "living will" helps clarify the wishes of the dying person as to the medical care they shall be given in the last stages of their life, even after they lose their discretion and reason. A donor card declares the willingness to donate organs after death, and advance medical directives may express the willingness to approve the use of reproductive cells postmortem. But are full discretion and understanding of the meaning of death truly present? What is the validity of a person's declaration that they wish to donate organs after their death? An even more basic question concerning the dead donor rule arises: to which definition of death does the informed consent refer? What is the nature of informed consent among those who are not aware of the dispute surrounding brain death? Furthermore, unlike consent to participate in an experiment or receive a specific medical treatment, in the case of postmortem organ donation, the donor cannot question the process itself or its results, which detracts from the right at the basis of the idea of informed consent. Another question is whether organ donation is equal to any other inheritance. Does a person have full ownership of their body after death in such a way that allows them to bequeath parts of it? Does the loss of control of our bodies after death not indicate the loss of self-sovereignty over the body? According to many religious views, a person's sovereignty over their body is limited to begin with (suicide in different faiths can serve as an example). Only a solid materialist view makes it possible to perceive the body as mere matter and, therefore, as something whose ownership can be determined. Such a view is just one item in the rich menu of cultural perspectives on the mind–body problem.

The third reason transplantation medicine challenges the idea of informed consent is perhaps the ultimate reason: consent to organ donation is not related to medical ethics or physician–patient relations. It is about an ethical gesture to society on deceased organ donation or to someone you care in living organ donations. In this perspective, consent to organ donation obtains a unique flare, distinct from conventional informed consent in medical ethics. In fact, consent to organ donation involves a notion of solidarity and awareness to the problem of organ shortage as a societal problem. Moreover, as an answer to the organ shortage, modalities of consent to organ donations are an exercise in public health ethics. The ethical question for public health policymakers is how to alleviate the burden of organ shortage on one side and preserve the principle of autonomy on the other side. Organ shortage is conceived in terms of motivating populations to become organ donors and it is another issue of public health. From that aspect, the policymakers' goal is the utmost reduction of the shortage while maintaining ethical rules, especially the rules related to motivation for donation. The wishes of the deceased and consent to donate are thereby combined into a single consideration in the totality of considerations in dealing with the shortage problem. But neither public health ethics nor liberal bioethics engages persuasively with the question of the wishes of the deceased on the philosophical level; both suppose a direct association between consent in life and the wishes of the deceased, even though that association is questionable.

In conclusion, the question of consent concerning the procurement and distribution of organs for transplantation has three dimensions. One dimension is the agreement of the living donor to donate an organ, and the patient's consent to undergo the transplant. In that dimension, the consent is based on the principles of autonomy and informed consent as they developed in liberal bioethics. The second dimension of the consent is signing a donor card, expressing the willingness to donate organs after death. In that dimension, informed consent is quite obscure and has more in common with the consent model in medicine before the development of liberal bioethics. The third dimension arises from attaching the consent question to the shortage question, which is perceived as a public health issue. In that dimension, the reference unit is the population, and the mission is to mobilize the public to donate organs. Here, consent is only a tactical matter, whereas the strategic goal is reducing the shortage. The nervous fluctuations in the consent policy from presumed consent to informed consent and vice versa are evidence of that, as can be seen from the dispute in France and the United Kingdom.

The turn to presumed consent, therefore, arises from a utilitarian consideration – the desire to reduce the shortage. And sure enough, this policy does, indeed, reduce the shortage, even if it does not completely overcome it (Arshad, Anderson and Sharif 2019). But presumed consent, or the presumption of consent, is also problematic, considering the public's incomplete knowledge of the definition of death and the organ donation process. Moreover, ethnographic studies show that models of presumed consent push strong populations out of the donor pool; meanwhile, disempowered populations, who are not even aware of the existence of the policy and have limited contact with the establishment, are perceived, often erroneously, as potential organ donors (Goodwin 2001). Therefore, the consent question does not provide a clear solution to the organ shortage problem.

Exercising ethics: organ markets and the altruistic code

The dead donor rule and consent policies have not managed to solve the shortage problem. In the 1990s, when transplantation medicine grew significantly, the problem only worsened, and the number of patients waiting for organs for transplantation shot up.[6] During that decade, after the introduction of immunosuppression agents, transplantation medicine was already considered routine medicine. It saved tens of thousands of lives worldwide and gave patients a good quality of life and long life expectancy. In fact, organ shortage remained since then as the main obstacle to the expansion of transplantation medicine. Organ shortage was conceived not only as a problem in the actual procurement of cadavers or living donor but also in the ethical framing that obliged donations to be altruistic. Opponents of the altruism model contend that introducing materialistic rewards to organ donation will help reducing the shortage problem (Taylor 2017, Cherry 2015, Matas 2004).

The altruistic code commands that organ donation would be without compensation: in its extreme form, it negates any monetary consideration. In its softer form, it allows compensating the living donor for any losses they may have suffered or giving them a nonmonetary compensation (Delmonico, Arnold and Youngner 2002, Gaston, Danovitch, Epstein et al. 2006). But the term "altruism" in itself does not appear in legislation or official definitions of motivation for donation and is only defined as the reverse of illegitimate motivations, especially financial incentives, or simply as voluntarism. As we shall see below, this negative definition of altruism – as what altruism is not – creates a problem of conceptualization.

Usually, altruism is referred as the voluntary, autonomous, free will of an individual to act toward an other individual, with an element of a personal cost or even self-sacrifice.[7] In the context of organ donation, the donation of one's bodily organs toward the benefit of an unknown stranger is regarded as meeting these general criteria of altruism. Nonetheless, the application of altruism to organ donation requires a nuanced definition when it comes to donation within family members that direct their donation to a specific person or in the case of post-mortem donation where it is the family who consent to donate their late relative organs. In fact, most of the organ donations introduce a soft version of altruism with each donation pattern presenting a different notion of altruism and voluntarism. With such diverse and sometime contradictory applications of altruism in organ donation, is there another role that altruism plays in the ethics of organ donation?

Altruism fosters the notion of consent by emphasizing its unconditional aspect. Altruism and consent, especially in its informed mode, go hand in hand in their emphasis on free will, autonomous, and materialistic-free motivation. The notion of altruism and voluntarism became dispensable to the ethics of transplantation. The altruism concept in transplant medicine focuses on the question of motivation to donate: it must be free of any ulterior motive that might violate the principle of informed consent. The combination of altruism and informed consent creates a uniform and coherent concept of a subject whose nobility derives from their Kantian wisdom and autonomy. Altruism, in fact, emphasizes what Kant saw as autonomy – a will that is free of any heteronomous intervention that is critical by its own right. This concept of autonomy stands at the heart of Kant's idea of the enlightened person and is an ethical challenge that is hard to meet. In its purest form, as a virtue that negates materialistic motivations, altruism fosters this notion of autonomy that stands at the heart of modern bioethics' concept of consent.

This concept of autonomy is a very well-defined concept historically, culturally, and politically and is the product of Western thought and politics. The abstraction of that autonomous subject and its transformation into a universal model is typical of Western philosophy and liberal bioethics and stands at its core. In this section, I will briefly examine the development of the altruistic code in transplant medicine from two aspects. First, I will check the relationship between altruism and the suggestions to establish organ markets to meet the shortage question. Second, I will look at the link between the altruistic concept and the dead donor rule, the question of the wishes of the deceased and informed consent.

The idea to establish organ markets was rejected out of hand by most of the countries in the world.[8] The reason is the moral problems involved in such markets, especially the trafficking in human organs and the damage such trafficking might cause (Danovitch 2014). An examination of the legislation in numerous countries and the international conventions that refer to organ transplants finds that payment for organs is the main ethical concern.[9] Human organs, as Margaret Radin argued in her seminal article "Market Inalienability," are not transferable or tradable (Radin 1987).[10] This view is salient in the 2008 Declaration of Istanbul on Organ Trafficking and Transplant Tourism, according to which any economic or material incentive for organ donation is an illegitimate manifestation of organ trafficking (Martin, Van Assche, Domínguez-Gil et al. 2019).[11] The Istanbul declaration is the result of years-long efforts to unify the condemnation of organ markets into a common ethical code, and it has a profound impact on legislation all over the world, fostering the status of altruism and voluntarism as the key motivation for organ donation.

Nonetheless, theoretical proposals to establish organ markets in different ways and on varying scales are raised constantly (Danovitch and Leichtman 2006, Harmon and Delmonico 2006). Supporters of the establishment of organ markets distinguish between state-regulated and supervised organ markets and illegal organ trafficking to unregulated organ markets (Kasserman and Barnett 2002). Regulated markets rely on a conception that any individual has the right to sell, even their own organs, in a free market. These perceptions insist on the individual's right to sell and buy organs based on their free will, as they do with any other product (Taylor 2017). Supporters of the organ market believe that the altruism principle is a barrier to finding a significant solution to the shortage problem. Replacing it by materialistic incentives – mainly money – will help in increasing the demand of organs. In fostering the idea of organ markets, proponents of that idea must first of all wrestle with the idea of altruism as a right motivation for massive organ procurement.[12]

The argument for organ markets stems from a utilitarian approach. Placing the organ shortage problem, supporters of organ markets claim that it cannot be solved by approaching the good heart of people. From a utilitarian point of view, altruism is simply not enough and cannot provide the huge amount of needed donations. However, the shortage cannot be attributed to the altruism principle alone; there are other factors that affect it, for instance, the decline in cases of brain death or logistic problems in detecting donation candidates and methods of transplant coordination (Thorne 1998). The fact that those who advocate organ markets pay little attention to other factors that exacerbate organ shortage may also have to do with the perception that once the ethical question is solved, other shortage determinants will also be resolved. This notion of "ethical determinism" – of both opponents and proponents of altruism – suggests that organ shortage depends on the ethical framing of the permitted and forbidden in organ donation.

But, the objection to establishing organ markets goes far beyond transplantation medicine, in general, and the question of the organ shortage, in particular. The notion of organ markets is in sharp contrast with well-rooted ethical and moral perceptions that negate commodification of body parts (Waldby and Cooper 2008). In the backdrop of modern capitalist societies, where utilitarianism and self-profit are the norms, this opposition strikes as at least strange. Economist and anthropologist Karl Polanyi's historical analysis of the emergence of the free market can help understand this apparent contradiction. Although transplant medicine was still science fiction in the 1940s, Polanyi's argument can help understand why bodily commodification is so provocative in our market-based societies. In his book *The Great Transformation* (1944), Polanyi analyses the counter-reaction to capitalism in the 1920s and the 1930s and the following introduction of totalitarian regimes in that time. These regimes, he argues, were counter-reactions to expanding practices of capitalism, liberalism, and the free market. Those regimes objected mainly to the commodification of land, labor, and money that were capitalized and circulated in the free markets as commodities. These are "fictitious commodities" because they are not produced like ordinary commodities and, therefore, their value is determined only in the abstract market context. Polanyi argued that the expansion of fictitious commodities aroused suspicion and resentment to the very idea of the abstract free market and "the invisible hand" principle. It raised doubt in free markets are equal and fair and contributed to the rise of political theories that undermine capitalism and liberalism.

Polanyi's warning that unbridled commodification of the free market undermines the foundations of society and can lead to the rise of totalitarianism resonates powerfully even today. Today's fictitious commodity is our body, its organs, tissues, and genetic composition (Dickenson 2017). The threat of this commodification is far-reaching, and organ trafficking is only one of its manifestations. Among other things, it concerns issues such as payment for egg donations and surrogacy, the question of ownership of economic assets related to body organs, and even the question of the economic value of knowledge stored in citizens' genetic databases (biobanks). Like the commodification of money, land, and labor and their transformation into the masters of capitalism, so does the commodification of body parts and genetic information elicit fierce antagonism. That is the context in which the broad resistance to organ markets and the development of the altruistic code as a preemptive measure should be examined. This is the reason organ trafficking became a metaphor for capitalism decadence and organ markets a controversial suggestion.

But, the altruistic code has a role not only in the objection to establishing organ markets. I argue it has another, more hidden, and perhaps not completely conscious function. That role has to do with the problems surrounding the dead donor rule and the question of informed consent and the wishes of the deceased, which were discussed above. We saw that informed consent to postmortem donation raises a logical question: it is hard to think about informed consent in unknown conditions such as death, mostly in the problematic definition of brain death; it is hard to think independently about a situation we have never experienced before and to express wishes concerning that situation. Consent to donate organs is at best simple consent, not informed consent. Are people who sign donor cards fully aware of the dispute over brain death – despite the medical and scientific consensus that it is absolute, or at least that it is an irreversible condition that leads to death? Are people fully informed of the particularities that differentiate cardiac from brain death and are they aware of the detailed protocol of defining such a death? As the dead donor rule determines, death is sine qua non of organ donation and without understanding what death means, consent – informed or presumed – is altogether problematic.

I claim that the altruism principle fills this gap. In altruism, the sacrifice made is not only of the donated organ but also of the problem of consent. When someone makes a conscious autonomous altruistic act, other considerations are at least marginalized if not erased. This is the idea of sacrificial altruism, this is "the cost" one pays in order to become altruistic. In our context, the problem of consent and the dead donor rule are marginalized in favor of the mere sacrifice. The altruist, strange as it may sound, is not bounded by any ethical rule. Altruism is beyond ethics; as a moral action, it surmounts ethical considerations.[13] The altruistic individuals holds the key to ethical problems by placing their sacrifice and goodwill above any other considerations.[14] While the surrounding professional experts that treat and determine the individual's death are obliged to conduct according to protocols and ethical frameworks, the altruist is free of such calculations. This makes his consent not necessarily informed but rather altruistic. Thus, "altruistic consent" removes the ethical difficulties of informed consent to brain death. The questions of responsibility and ethics are absorbed by the very altruistic action, the reduction of the self for the well-being of the other. They are no longer anchored in external ethical frameworks but rather become inherent to that action.

A complimentary function to the "altruistic consent" is found in organ donations by living people. Altruism absolves the doctor from the commitment to the primal ethical rule of "first do no harm." The damage of extracting a kidney or other organ from the body of a healthy person in order to cure another person may be justified by utilitarian standards: the damage to the donor is much less than the benefit to the recipient. But, that argument alone is not enough to completely cancel that rule, which requires altruism because the act of sacrifice inherent in the concept of altruism neutralizes the concept of damage. In fact, altruism is all about "the cost" one pays for the benefit of another. Moreover, the value of sacrifice is engraved in the Judeo-Christian culture, in which transplantation medicine arose. Furthermore, sacrifice is consistent with the principle of autonomy in bioethics and even raises it to a higher level, where in the name of that principle individuals are allowed to perform acts of altruism even if they thereby harm themselves.[15]

Despite the considerable efforts invested in the attempt to solve the problem of organ supply and the shortage of organs for transplantation, the problem only exacerbated over the years. Alongside the remarkable progress in transplant medicine, an ethics of shortage is developing. Concepts such as the dead donor rule, brain death, or altruism as well as policy changes of opt-in or opt-out are the building blocks of organ shortage ethics. But from where I stand, the history of transplant ethics is intellectually fascinating but personally frustrating. It seems that these exercises in shortage do not reach a solution. Maybe there is not a solution? Perhaps organ transplantations carry with them a baggage of cultural taboos, fears, and concerns that policies and regulation just can't dissolve? The next chapter tackles this question by exploring two contradictory cultural narratives of transplant medicine. One frames transplantations as dystopia, the other as utopia. In lieu of them, I will argue for a third narrative.

Notes

1 Donations after circulatory death (DCD) increased to 2130 from 1883 in 2018; this number has been increasing since 2007. The number of organs authorized for recovery from actual deceased donors continued to increase, to 77,012 in 2018 from 73,638 in 2017; this number has been increasing since 2010. The number of organs recovered for transplant and transplanted increased to 30,595 in 2018 from 29,435 in 2017. For more, see Israni, Zaun, Hadley et al. (2020).

2 The data is as of July 2018. See: National Kidney Foundation, "End Stage Renal Disease in the United States" (online).

3 These criteria were updated throughout the years. For a rather recent protocol, see Spinello (2015).

4 For the 50th anniversary to brain death definition in 2018, the Hastings Center Report issued a collection of essays delineating brain death's history and controversies ("Defining Death: Organ Transplantation and the Fifty-Year Legacy of the Harvard Report on Brain Death" Volume 48 (S4) November–December 2018). See, for example, Truog and Berlinger (2018).

5 Some of his main arguments throuout the years are in Veatch 2000, 1992, 1975, 1972).

6 See Figures 1.1 and 1.2.

7 Leaving conceptualization of altruism in sociobiology aside, one can find a wide discussion on altruism as a virtue in moral philosophy (Nagel 1978 as the most prominent example). Accounts on altruism from sociology, economics, and psychology draw a nuanced notion of altruism where one can find altruism as embedded in social relations of reciprocity, competition, and cooperation. See Fehr and Schmidt (2006).

8 Iran is the exception where a regulated markets for organs (mainly kidneys) replaced unregulated and black market. The state-governed market was created as an answer for organ shortage. For more on Iran's organ procurement policy, see Chapter 4 and Fry-Revere (2014), and Mahdavi-Mazdeh (2012).

9 On March 2011, The Council of the European Union adopted supplementing the definition of criminal offenses and the level of sanctions in order to strengthen the prevention of organ trafficking. See also report of the European Parliament of organ trafficking: https://www.europarl.europa.eu/RegData/etudes/STUD/2015/549055/EXPO_STU%282015%29549055_EN.pdf.

10 See Radin (1987).

11 International summit on organ trafficking. 2008. The declaration of Istanbul on organ trafficking and transplant tourism. *Clinical Journal of American Society of Nephrology* 20083(5):1227–1231. See an updated version of the declaration from 2018 at issue 103 of the journal "Transplantation" volume 2, pp. 218–219. See also: Martin, Van Assche, Domínguez-Gil et al. (2019).

12 As legal scholar Glenn Cohen suggests, the altruistic code is the organizing axis of the moral economy of organ transplantation, from which arguments for and against organ markets depart. See Cohen (2003).

13 This is not to say that someone who objects to brain death cannot be altruist, but that in its ultimate form altruism solves the dead donor rule and the problem of consent. When conditioning the donation upon a critical scrutiny of their death determination than both consent, voluntarism and good will exist. But, the detailed condition renders this altruism more softer.

14 In the most significant way, altruists may also sacrifice their own life for saving the other. For example, stories of soldiers jumping onto explosive grenade. There is no military training that instruct soldier to do so, but when such an altruistic self-sacrifice act occurs, the most distinguished recognition is granted. For more on this, see Hubner and Hauser (2011).

15 It is important to note that the altruistic subject according to the classic model is not only autonomous but also universal. Both the self and the other are universal entities disconnected from local contexts. However, the autonomy of the altruistic subject may, in certain conditions, give rise precisely to a particular altruism. I will analyze these conditions when discussing the Israeli case.

References

Abadie, A., & Gay, S. (2006). The impact of presumed consent legislation on cadaveric organ donation: A cross-country study. *Journal of Health Economics*, 25(4), 599–620.

Abt, P. L., Desai, N. M., Crawford, M., Forman, L. M., Markmann, J. W., Olthoff, K. M., & Markmann, J. F. (2004). Survival following liver transplantation from non-heart-beating donors. *Annals of Surgery*, 239(1), 87–92.

Alexander, S. (1962). They decide who lives, who dies. *Life*, 53(19), 102–124.

Annas, G. J. (1988). The paradoxes of organ transplantation. *American Journal of Public Health*, 78(6), 621–622.

Arshad, A., Anderson, B., & Sharif, A. (2019). Comparison of organ donation and transplantation rates between opt-out and opt-in systems. *Kidney International*, 95(6), 1453–1460.

Beecher, H. K. (1968). Ethical problems created by the unconscious patient. *New England Journal of Medicine*, 278(26), 1425–1430.

Belkin, G. (2014). *Death before Dying: History, Medicine and Brain Death*, Oxford: Oxford University Press.

Belkin, G. (2003). Brain death and the historical understanding of bioethics. *Journal of the History of Medicine and Allied Sciences*, 58(3), 325–361.

Bernat, J. L., Culver, C. M., & Gert, B. (1981). On the definition and criterion of death. *Medicine and Public Issues*, 94, 389–394.

Bernat, J. L. (1992). How much of the brain must die in brain death? *Journal of Clinical Ethics*, 3(1), 21–26.

Beauchamp, T. (2004). "Informed consent", in S. G. Post, (ed). *Encyclopedia of Bioethics*, 5 Volume Set, Thomson Gale/Macmillan, 1271–1313.

Beauchamp, T. L., & Childress, J. F. (2001). *Principles of Biomedical Ethics*. USA: Oxford University Press.

Blagg, C. R. (1999). The early years of chronic dialysis: The seattle contribution. *American Journal of Nephrology*, 19(2), 350–354.

Capron, A. M. (2001). Brain death—Well settled yet still unresolved. *New England Journal of Medicine*, 344(16), 1244–1246.

Cherry, M. J. (2015). *Kidney for Sale by Owner: Human Organs, Transplantation and the Market*, Washington: Georgetown University Press.

Childress, J. F. (1970). Who shall live when not all can live? *Soundings*, 53(4), 339–355.

Cohen, I. G. (2003). The price of everything, the value of nothing: reframing the commodification debate. *Harvard Law Review*, 117, 689.

Cook, P. J., & Krawiec, K. D. (2014). A primer on kidney transplantation: Anatomy of the shortage. *Law and Contemporary Problems*, 77(3), 1–23.

Danovitch, G. (2014). The high cost of organ transplant tourism. *Kidney International*, 85(2), 248–250.

Danovitch, G. M., & Leichtman, A. B. (2006). Kidney vending: The "Trojan horse" of organ transplantation. *Clinical Journal of the American Society of Nephrology*, 1(6), 1133–1135.

Darrah, J. B. (1987). The committee. *ASAIO Journal*, 33(4), 791–793.

Delmonico, F. L., Arnold, R., & Youngner, S. J. (2002). Ethical incentives—Not payment—For organ donation. *The New England Journal of Medicine*, 346, 25.

Dickenson, D. (2017). *Property in the Body*, Cambridge: Cambridge University Press.

Fehr, E., & Schmidt, K. M. (2006). The economics of fairness, reciprocity and altruism—Experimental evidence and new theories. *Handbook of the Economics of Giving, Altruism and Reciprocity*, 1, 615–691.

Fox, R. C., & Swazey, J. P. (1974). *The Courage to Fail: A Social View of Organ Transplants and Dialysis*, Piscataway, NJ: Transaction Publishers.

Fry-Revere, S. (2014). *The Kidney Sellers – A Journey of Discovery in Iran*, Durham, NC: Carolina Academic Press.

Gaston, R. S., Danovitch, G. M., Epstein, R. A., Kahn, J. P., Matas, A. J., & Schnitzler, M. A. (2006). Limiting financial disincentives in live organ donation: A rational solution to the kidney shortage. *American Journal of Transplantation*, 6(11), 2548–2555.

Geneau, R., Stuckler, D., Stachenko, S. et al. (2010). Raising the priority of preventing chronic diseases: A political process. *The Lancet*, 376(9753), 1689–1698.

Giacomini, M. (1997). A change of heart and a change of mind? Technology and the redefinition of death in 1968. *Social Science & Medicine*, 44(10): 1465–1482.

Goodwin, M. (2001). Deconstructing legislative consent law: Organ taking, racial profiling and distributive justice. *Virginia Journal of Law and Technology*, 6, 1.

Gray, F. D. (1998). *The Tuskegee Syphilis Study: The Real Story and Beyond*, Montgomery, AL: NewSouth Books.

Harmon, W., & Delmonico, F. (2006). Payment for kidneys: A government-regulated system is not ethically achievable. *Clinical Journal of the American Society of Nephrology*, 1(6), 1146–1147.

Hubner, B., & Hauser, M. D. (2011). Moral judgements about altruistic self-sacrifice: When philosophical and folk institutions clash. *Philosophical Psychology*, 24 (1), 73–94.

Israni, A. K., Zaun, D., Hadley, N. et al. (2020). OPTN/SRTR 2018 Annual Data Report: Deceased organ donation. *American Joiurnal of Transplantation*. https://doi.org/10.1111/ajt.15678

Jonsen, A. R. (1998). *The Birth of Bioethics*, New York: Oxford: Oxford University.

Kaserman, D. L., & Barnett, A. H. (2002). *The US Organ Procurement System: A Prescription for Reform*, Washington, DC: American Enterprise Institute.

Keizer, K. M., De Fijter, J. W., Haase-Kromwijk, B., & Weimar, W. (2005). Non–heart-beating donor kidneys in The Netherlands: Allocation and outcome of transplantation. *Transplantation*, 79(9), 1195–1199.

Mahdavi-Mazdeh, M. (2012). The Iranian model of living renal transplantation. *Kidney International*, 82(6), 627–634.

Martin, D. E., Van Assche, K., Domínguez-Gil, B., López-Fraga, M., Garcia Gallont, R., Muller, E., Rondeau, E., and Capron, A. M. (2019). A new edition of the declaration of Istanbul: Updated guidance to Combat organ trafficking and transplant tourism world-wide. *Kidney International*, 95(4), 757–759.

Matas, A. J. (2004). The case for living kidney sales: Rationale, objections and concerns. *American Journal of Transplantations*, 4(12), 2007–2017.

Nagel, T. (1978). *The Possibility of Altruism*, Princeton, NJ: Princeton University Press.

Pernick, M. S. (1999). "Brain death in a cultural context", in S. Youngner, R. M. Arnold, & R. Schapiro (eds). *The Definition of Death: Contemporary Controversies*, Baltimore and London: Johns Hopkins University Press. pp. 3–33.

Polanyi, K. (1944). *The Great Transformation*, Boston: Beacon.

Radin, M. J. (1987). Market-inalienability. *Harvard Law Review*, 100(8), 1849–1937.

Rescher, N. (1969). The allocation of exotic medical lifesaving therapy. *Ethics*, 79(3), 173–186.

Rizvi, S. A. H., Naqvi, Z. H., Zafar, H. et al. (2003). Renal transplantation in developing countries. *Kidney International*, 63(83), S96–S100.

Robertson, J. A. (1999). Delimiting the donor: The dead donor rule. *Hastings Center Report*, 29(6), 6–14.

Ross, L. F., & Thistlethwaite, J. R. (2016). The 1966 Ciba symposium on transplantation ethics: 50 years later. *Transplantation*, 100(6), 1191–1197.

Sanders, D., & Dukeminier, J. (1967). Medical advance and legal lag: Hemodialysis and kidney transplantation. *UCLA Law Review*, 15, 357.

Schreiner, G. E. (1966). *Problems of Ethics in Relation to Haemo-Dialysis and Transplanta-tion. Ciba Foundation Symposium-Ethics in Medical Progress: With Special Reference to Transplantation*, Chichester: Wiley Online Library.

Sheehy, E., Suzanne, L., Conrad, S. L. et al. (2003). Estimating the number of potential organ donors in the United States. *New England Journal of Medicine*, 349(7), 667–674.

Spinello, I. M. (2015). Brain death determination. *Journal of Intensive Care Medicine*, 30(-6), 326–337.

Starzl, T. E. (1992). *The Puzzle People: Memoirs of a Transplant Surgeon*, Pittsburgh, PA: University of Pittsburgh Press.

Steinbrook, R. (2007). Organ donation after cardiac death. *New England Journal of Med-icine*, 357(3), 209–213.

Taylor, J. S. (2017). *Stakes and Kidneys: Why Markets in Human Bodies are Morally Impera-tive*, London & New York: Routledge.

Thorne, E.D. (1998). The shortage in market-inalienable human organs: A consideration of "Nonmarket" failures. *American Journal of Economics and Sociology*, 57(3), 247–260.

Truog, R. D., Berlinger. N., Zacharias, R. L., & Solomon, M. Z. (2018). Brain death at fifty: Exploring consensus, controversy, and contexts. *The Hastings Center Report*, 48, S4, 2–5.

Truog, R. D. & Robinson, W. M. (2003). Role of brain death and the dead-donor rule in the ethics of organ transplantation. *Critical Care Medicine*, 31(9), 2391–2396.

Truog, R. D., & Miller, F. G. (2008). The dead donor rule and organ transplantation. *New England Journal of Medicine*, 359(7), 674–675.

Usman, A., Afif, H., Ahmed-Zayn, M. et al. (2019). A systematic review of opt-out versus opt-in consent on deceased organ donation and transplantation (2006–2016). *World Journal of Surgery*, 43(12), 3161–3171.

Veatch, R. M. (2018). Would a reasonable person now accept the 1968 Harvard brain death report? A short history of brain death. *Hastings Center Report*, 48, S4, 6–9.

Veatch, R. M. (2000). *Transplantation Ethics*, Washington: Georgetown University Press.

Veatch, R. M. (1992). Brain death and slippery slopes. *Journal of Clinical Ethics*, Fall; 3(3), 181–187.

Veatch, R. M. (1975). The whole-brain-oriented concept of death: An outmoded philosophical formulation. *Journal of Thanatology*, 3(1), 13–30.

Veatch, R. M. (1972). Brain death: Welcome definition... Or dangerous judgment? *Hastings Center Report*, 2(5), 10–13.

Waldby, C., & Cooper, M. (2008). The biopolitics of reproduction: Post-Fordist biotechnology and women's clinical labour. *Australian Feminist Studies*, 23(55), 57–73.

Youngner, S.J. (2003). Some must die. *Zygon*, 38(3), 705–724.

Youngner, S. J., Arnold, R. M., & Schapiro, R. (eds.). (2002). *The Definition of Death: Contemporary Controversies*, Baltimore and London: Johns Hopkins University Press.

2 The Making of Utopia and Dystopia in Organ Transplantations

A mystified discourse

The possibility of replacing a failed organ with a healthy one, dividing the body into its constituent parts, reassembling it, and thereby creating a state of health in the diseased body has been fueling medicine's imagination and fantasies for many years. The transplantation of organs has been accorded a symbolic role in the history of medicine: it represented both the endpoint of the realia of the medical act and the beginning of the fantastic (Morris 2004, Tilney 2003, Bergan 1997). The Minotaur, Chimera, and the Sphinx are products of cross-breeding, combinations of species that in their monstrousness testify that hybridization, the mixing of incompatible things, the creation of a species not of its kind, is not given into human hands but is a supernatural act. In view of medicine's failures in transplant surgery over the years, this attempt to exceed the purview of human beings came to be considered hubris. Medicine, both eastern and western, is thus ruled by the anthropomorphic axiom that man is trapped within his own skin. The body holds absolute sway – one person, one body, one life. Deviations from this anthropomorphic axiom have been – and perhaps still are – a violation of natural law; by their very unnaturalness, they herald either divine revelation or a satanic event. The miraculous grafting of a corpse's leg onto a Christian's body ascribed to the martyrs Damian and Cosmas, twin brothers who practiced medicine, led to their execution at the beginning of the 4th century C.E. The creation of humanoids by means of the transference, grafting, and joining of organs has been viewed as something wondrous, perhaps satanic or perhaps God-like, but certainly not something vouchsafed to human hands. Therefore, only the flesh of the Christian messiah can become realized time after time in the Catholic mass, and therefore only God Himself can promise, "And I will give them one heart, and I will put a new spirit within them; and I will take the stony heart out of their flesh, and will give them a heart of flesh" (Ezekiel 11:19).

However, even now that the fantastic has become reality as transplant surgery has become routine, the language of metaphors, imagery, figurative idioms, and symbolism still holds us captive, remaining the accepted discourse to refer to organ transplants. The body as a "repository of parts" and organs as "spare parts" are commonplace images in speech and writing about organ transplants. But is

DOI: 10.4324/9781003288886-3

this merely imagery, or a realistic description? In point of fact, an inventory of the organs that can be taken from the donor's body (the heart, pancreas, liver, two lungs, two kidneys, and more recently intestines) does suggest an association with a repository and spare parts, but using these images loads the act of transplantation with a meaning that diminishes the donor's humanity to nothing more than a body of objects. In this way, a negative association with the act of transplantation is created.

In contrast, the expression "the gift of life" is an empowering image; it provides a heroic significance of the giving of life, similar to birth or the merit of miraculous healing ascribed to saints, angels, and kings. "The gift of life" presents organ donation in terms of heroism and generosity; the wonder of a life-giving gift elevates the donor to a veritably divine level.

Organs as mere objects or organs as the potential bearers of "the gift of life"? An affront to human dignity or the glorification of the noblest of acts? Even if we take both options as they relate to various aspects of organ transplantation, these aspects are saturated with metaphoric language. Figurative language serves to frame the universe of transplantation, whether by praise or condemnation. The realia itself, in a manner of speaking, become subservient to images that fluctuate between diminution and elevation. Metaphoric language evolves into a language of morality. The moral aspect is interwoven with the language of imagery, now elevating the analogy to a super-human level ("the gift of life"), now lowering it to a sub-human one ("spare parts repository"). To find intermediate levels is difficult. The transplantation of organs is presented to us as a duality. It may praise or it may condemn; one of its manifestations reveals a macabre setting full of gothic, Faustian hints of deviant medicine, while its antithesis comprises themes of heroism, community, nobility of spirit, and immortality. Transplant medicine appears as an allegory for moral decay or alternately for moral transcendence. Metaphoric language, thus, directs us toward dual judgments: altruism, kindness, and generosity, or utilitarianism, exploitation, and the objectification of the body. Each choice within the semantic field is, in fact, an act in the universe of morality: "the gift of life" or "a spare parts repository" – to continue with the previous examples – enfolds within it a pronouncement, glorifying or diminishing, about organ transplantation.

This chapter examines the underpinning epistemology of dystopic and utopic narratives on organ transplantations. For exploring a dystopic narrative, I will present the discourse of medical anthropologists that accompanied the inception and development of transplant medicine from the last quarter of the last century up until the first years of this millennium. For introducing a utopian narrative, I will investigate the cultural roots of the "gift of life" discourse. In the previous chapter, the shortcomings of the ethical discourse about organ shortage were presented. In this chapter, I wish to explore the moralist biases of the dualistic images of transplant medicine. Together, these chapters pave the way for an analysis that is more reflective to the partialities of the transplant discourse both in the popular stage and in the academic literature, mainly of medical anthropology.

Dystopia – transplants as moral decay

In 1992, the anthropologist Susan DiGiacomo paraphrased Susan Sontag's "illness as metaphor," rendering it instead "metaphor as illness" (DiGiacomo 1992). Her argument is that the metaphor has been transformed to become the illness of critical medical anthropology. Critical anthropology has been taken captive within the very language of images and analogies that it produced, creating confusion by fusing analytical concepts and symbolic language. Critical anthropological discourse about organ transplantation is dominated by figurative language, imagery, allegorical idioms, and metaphors. As such, it evokes an image of transplant medicine that renders it a symbol of moral decay.

A reading of ethnographies concerning organ transplants written during the development of transplants as experimental medicine in the 1970s and its institutionalization as a routine medicine from the 1990s to the early 2000s illustrates the truth of this assertion. Indeed, organ transplantations fascinate the anthropological imagination; It is not only the living organ of the dead donor, or the physiological redefinition of "self" and "other," and it is not just the challenge to the very concept of the individual (in-dividum), or the shifting boundaries of body and soul; object and subject – but the extent of it all that turn organ transplantations as provocation to anthropology's basic object of investigation – the ontology of mankind. With its ability to generate separate spheres, where body parts live outside their original bodies, transplantation technologies challenge the basic anthropomorphic assumption of one person, one body, one life and require us to rethink the anthropological assumption about the living body, self, and other as distinct concepts. Transplant medicine, thus, introduces classical anthropological questions in a guise of high-tech modern medicine. It became a lurid research site for the medical anthropologist who now has, at hand, what seems to be a clear case for articulating a new the ontology of life and death in modern societies. In what follows I will unfold the observations of medical anthropologists on the field of transplant medicine, written from a critical theory perspective. As critical theorists, medical anthropologists located transplant medicine in the context of modern biomedicine, capitalism, and science criticism. To a large extent, this point of view ceased to be hegemonic in medical anthropology writings on transplants in the last 15 years.

Two analytical axes characterize the critical writing about organ transplantation: the emphasis on the transplanted body as a metaphor and the observation that transplant medicine is a clear expression of medicalization. The combination of these interpretive axes leads to a view of transplantation as a sign that medicine has gone too far and is running wild. Renee Fox and Judith Swazey – historians and bio-ethicists of transplants, who became the uncontested competent authorities in medical anthropology, in general, and in the anthropology of organ transplants, in particular – provide a striking example of this perception in their book *Spare Parts* when they describe the universe of organ transplants:

> Organ replacement … has brought our society closer to the world of "rebuilt people" classically portrayed in science fiction, in which humans are more

and more composed of transplanted parts of one another, and of "man-machine unions" that prosthetize humans and humanize man-made organs.

Later in the same paragraph, they turn organ transplantation into an allegory of moral decay:

> It is the "spare parts" pragmatism, the vision of the "replaceable body" and limitless medical progress, and the escalating ardor about the life-saving goodness of repairing and remaking people in this fashion that we have found especially disturbing.
>
> (Fox and Swazey 1992:xv)

Swazey and Fox decided to leave the field of research and not to write further about organ transplantation. The above quotations are taken from a section that has become a classic in anthropological writing, representing researchers that take an ethical stand vis-à-vis the field. This is undoubtedly a dramatic step: there is nothing routine about a researcher abandoning his field of research in disgust, as Fox and Swazey do:

> Our decision to leave this field…is due not only to the cumulative participant-observer 'burnout' we have experienced. It is also motivated by our deepening social and moral concerns about the increasing zeal with which the procurement and transplantation of human organs and the quest to develop and implant artificial ones is being pursued. Allowing American medicine and the society of which it is a part to become too caught up in repairing and rebuilding people through organ replacement—while health care continues to be defined as a private consumption rather than a social good in American society, and while millions of people do not have adequate or even minimally decent care—speaks to a values framework and a vision of medical progress we find medically and morally untenable
>
> (ibid.)

One can understand Fox and Swazey's general aversion to the technique of organ transplantation against the backdrop of inequality in health insurance and access to medical technologies within the framework of the American health system. Yet, when their book was published in 1992, organ transplantation was not the same experimental medicine, with a limited target population that sanctified the technique of "rebuilding people" at great medical and personal cost to the transplanted patients that it was in the 1960s and 1970s. In the 1980s and 1990s, transplantation has become a routine medical procedure in a growing number of countries. In the United States alone, more than 16,000 transplants were performed in 1992.[1] It is reasonable to assume that Fox and Swazey were familiar with the data, but the metaphors of "rebuilt people," of "puzzle people" comprising organs taken from other people, forge a figurative dimension of the technique of organ transplants from which it is hard to break free.

Fox and Swazey's concern and distrust toward organ transplants have developed over long years of research in this field. Their collaboration in the area of organ transplantation began in the late 1960s, and throughout the 1970s, the two published *The Courage to Fail* (1974), in which they criticized medical transplantation and dialysis treatments as a kind of heroic medicine, that is, medicine that celebrates technological progress while being blind to the social, cultural, and personal harm that it causes. *The Courage to Fail* joins other critical writing that presents Western medicine as harmful (Illich 1976, Jonas 1974, 1969). According to this approach, man becomes dependent on medical technology, which not only fails to improve his chances of staying alive or the quality of his life but also forestalls any alternative to Western medicine. These processes of medicalization diminish our ability to look beyond the horizon demarcated by Western medicine and to comprehend life and death, health and sickness as primarily cultural concepts (Postman 2011, Cassell 1993, Ellul 1990). *The Courage to Fail* makes use of the transplants and dialysis treatments of the 1960s and early 1970s to promote their demonstration of the processes of medicalization. The claim that emerges is clear: the grueling dialysis treatments and the inability to improve and lengthen the lives of organ recipients present a further instance of the bondage of the concepts of health and illness, life and death to a medical technology that seemed, in the 1970s, to be but a dubious success. It should be said in their defense that, indeed, during the 1960s and 1970s, before the revolution that led to the body's successful acceptance of the implant by the suppression of the immune system, transplant medicine was truly experimental. *The Courage to Fail*, then, was in its time a call to curb this medicine described as running wild morally in its striving for technological mastery.

Swazey and Fox question the motives and the contribution of transplantation. During the years that they investigated this medicine, they were witness to many successes and many failures that accompanied this nascent medical specialty. Swazey and Fox criticized American consumerist society's system of norms that allowed transplantation medicine to thrive. From their standpoint, organ transplants and dialysis treatments are one more stage in the processes of the medicalization of the body, concepts of health and personal welfare. The main thrust of their criticism centers around what they see as society's inability to resist the momentum of Western medicine. Swazey and Fox counter these forces of medicalization with "the social view." This is a critical view, their rebuttal to what they consider the nullification of humanness by the machine, dialysis, and experiments – admittedly abortive in part – in the early 1970s to replace organs. Swazey and Fox formulate the dominant note in the critical discourse about organ transplants, inspiring generations of writers on the subject. For example, in 2006, the anthropologist Lesley Sharp addressed the decision by Swazey and Fox to abandon the field as a significant step in the anthropological investigation of organ transplants, and at the end of her book *Strange Harvest* (2006), she writes that the problems have only intensified since the publication of *Spare Parts* in the early 1990s. She adds, "If we expand the field to include the full range of activities that define organ transfer, we encounter still other developments that challenge the researcher's ability to maintain the impartiality assumed central to ethnographic inquiry" (Sharp 2006:243).

Admittedly, the tendency to use metaphoric language exists generally throughout anthropology. Although the anthropologists Nancy Scheper-Hughes and Margaret Lock (1987, 1986) propose the interpretive perspective as the central axis of analysis for medical anthropology, they continue a long tradition in the social sciences and humanities, in general, and in anthropology, in particular, that emphasizes the body as a metonymic system of social order. The phenomenology of the body and the emphasis on body image are translated in the research field of critical medical anthropology into what may be seen as "methodological symbolism" – the understanding of concepts of health and sickness by means of the symbolic dimension ascribed to health, disease, and the body.

In the framework of this method, diseases are social projects, and as such, they are immersed in symbolic meanings. Concepts of health and sickness are supported by cultural and philosophical interpretive frameworks determined by historical constellations. In other words, they consider the disease a metaphor; i.e., we provide meaning to the nature of the disease that has taken hold of us, to how we cope, and to the separation we make between health and sickness. The definition of a disease is therefore a function of time, culture, and place. In fact, this paradigm stands in contrast with the scientific perception in medicine that sees diseases as first and foremost physiological manifestations, based in large measure on the Cartesian dualism of the body as separate from the mind (Kleinman 1995). In contradistinction to the materialism and positivism of biomedicine, methodological symbolism proposes penetrating the iron curtain of positivism and replacing the rigidity of biomedicine with exposing the means of the disease's representation, emphasizing the social construction feature of diseases. Hence, methodological symbolism directs the researcher to interpretation, exposure of the multiplicity of facets, abstractions, images, allegories, and analogies used to express health and sickness.

Against the backdrop of the medical model, which reduces the complexity of body–society–culture–mind relations to mere biological models of physiological pathology, the alternative offered by methodological symbolism is a relativistic fashion of social construction. The self-evident analytical tool mandates focusing on the question of representation, the textualization of the body, and the symbolism that attaches to whether one makes his appearance in the world as healthy or sick. This is, in fact, an analytical process that is the opposite of that sought by Susan Sontag in her "illness as a metaphor" (1977). Instead of cleansing the disease of the metaphorical burden in which it is immersed, Scheper-Hughes and Lock argue that the disease is always a metaphor. It is nothing other than the representation of a perception, a view, of power relations. As such, separating the disease from its attendant metaphor is perceived as a futile process. Cleansing the disease of metaphorical thinking, according to Scheper-Hughes and Lock, is tantamount to stripping away its humanness; after all, there is no body without its cultural subtext.

Consistent with this analytical framework, writings about organ transplants are rife with body images. The body, according to Scheper-Hughes and Lock's view, is the screen on which cultural perceptions of organ transplants are projected. Thus, ethnographies about organ transplantation deal with the dialectic of the body and the changing self (Gill and Lowes 2008, Sanner 2001, Sharp 1995), with images of the commoditized body (Scheper-Hughes 2002, Sharp 2001, 2000), or even with the body combating the rejection of the implant (Joralemon 1995).

Lesley Sharp notes the importance of imagery in her ethnographical research on the cultural construction of organ transplantation in the United States. Sharp argues that transplantation medicine is saturated with contradictions and cultural dissonances that only a richness of language can put right. Indeed, the tension between concepts of the self and the other, the living organ taken from the dead body, the gift of life, and the commodity, is the central axis of the discourse about organ transplantation. Sharp finds the various images principally among the transplant recipients. Transplantation according to Sharp has changed the concept of the self to include organs belonging to the other, resulting in the changing or expanded self. This is an internal mental process that changes the transplant recipient's concept of the self:

> This is not a simple process. The profusion of culturally generated metaphors that surround transplantation are evidence of this struggle. Recipients must respond to cultural notions of transplants as "unnatural acts" by embellishing this social process with powerful metaphors.… But transplant specialists run interference, for they are loathe to encourage such symbolic thinking. They insist that recipients—unlike donors—must depersonalize their organs. Oddly, such an attitude insists that bodies of the (post) industrial age (cf. Helman 1988) are better off reified: they are specialized machines.… Transplant personnel…are ignorant of the richness of experience that arises from the gestalt of organ-donor-recipient. Instead, they view the personalization or humanization of the organ as a sign of pathology, and as evidence that the recipient may require psychological counseling.
>
> (Sharp 1995:381)

Sharp finds the metaphorical language among the transplant recipients. She stresses the tension between the cultural construction of the transplanted organs as marking humanness among the recipients and their construction among the medical staff as marking physiological functionality. In a later study, Sharp points out the tension between the naturalistic perception nurtured by the medical transplantation staff and the imagery-rich perception found in the public discourse about organ transplants (Sharp 2006). An understanding of illness as a cultural construction certainly sunders the dualism of nature versus culture and the dominance of the physiological factor in the patterns of disease. But in limiting metaphorical language to a mere strategy of the recipients, Sharp ignores the enduring existence of organ transplants as an image or allegory in the very social research in which she herself is also a participant. She does not see how metaphorical language can trickle from the field of the research to that of the researchers themselves, from the *–emic* to the *–etic*. On occasion, she exercises caution with the images she uses in describing her research field, and sometimes, she is tempted into using metaphorical language herself. The condemnation found more extensively among Sharp's counterparts is somewhat blunted in her work. In other words, it is not only the recipients who need metaphors to bridge the dissonances that become apparent in the very act of organ transplantation itself; the researchers also need the language of imagery to satisfy exactly the same need.

Organ transplantation as organ trafficking: the conflation of the metaphoric, the political, and the moral

When symbolism reaches an overflow point, the distinction between the emic and the etic is blurred and images and metaphors become the tools of both description and analysis. Medical anthropologists have transformed organ transplantation from being the object of research to being an image, a vessel for thinking about something else, or in short, a metaphor. The excess resort to the language of imagery is found more extensively and strikingly in the anthropology of organ trafficking, where methodological symbolism, despite the criticism of scientific positivism that it suggests, spins dizzyingly to the point of an unclear mixture of images and metaphors. This is somewhat strange, since in organ trafficking the political critique is somewhat straightforward without any need for semantic scaffoldings. Nonetheless, it is in the anthropological writings on organ trafficking where we find a conspicuous instance of the obscuring of the boundary between image as an analytical tool and image as a research object. The obscuring is done consciously. It is part of an ideological tool critical of the division between object and subject, researcher and what is being studied, context and content, and the universe of fact and that of fiction.

Nancy Scheper-Hughes is one of the most influential anthropologists in the area of the social research of organ transplantation although her main research was conducted in the late 1990s and in the 2000s. To a great extent, she continues the research program outlined by Fox and Swazey: organ transplants as an instance of carrying medicalization to the extreme, as a conspicuous example of combining capitalism and medicine manifest in the commercialization of the body. But while Swazey and Fox concentrated primarily on criticism of medicalization and on what they considered medical hubris, Scheper-Hughes focuses mainly on transplantation's social implications in an era of globalization and a neo-liberal economy. In Scheper-Hughes' view, in the age of a global economy, transplantation represents two examples of unfettered imperialism: the imperialism of medicine and of capitalism. The first relates to medicalization and the second, to commercialization of the body – in other words, to organ trafficking. In 2000, Scheper-Hughes published a panoramic article in the journal *Current Anthropology* in which she reviewed a collection of ethnographies on the subject of the globalization of organ trafficking, which she compiled together with her collaborators (Scheper-Hughes 2000). She also published similar summaries in the years that followed (Scheper-Hughes 2001, 2002, 2003), but the 2000 text is central, both because the journal chose to publish comments and reactions along with her paper and because it presents Scheper-Hughes' personal credo regarding the role of critical anthropology in the study of transplantation medicine. At the beginning of the article, Scheper-Hughes raises questions about the most suitable analytical framework for this field of study. Her conclusion embraces the interpretive axes noted above, criticism of processes of medicalization, horrifying body images as a metaphor for social order, and a critique of processes of globalization:

> But perhaps what is needed from anthropology is something more akin to Donna Haraway's radical manifesto for the cyborg bodies and cyborg selves that we have already become. The emergence of strange markets, excess capital, "surplus bodies," and spare body parts has generated a global body trade which promises select individuals of reasonable economic means living almost anywhere in the world—from the Amazon Basin to the deserts of Oman—a miraculous extension of what Giorgio Agamben refers to as *bios*—brute or naked life, the elementary form of species life. In the face of this late-modern dilemma—this particular "end of the body"—the task of anthropology is relatively straightforward: to activate our discipline's radical epistemological promise and our commitment to the primacy of the ethical.
> (Scheper-Hughes 2000:193)

It seems to me that this paragraph, with its theoretical load (Haraway, Agamben) and language of sensation ("spare body parts," "surplus bodies"), clearly and thoroughly covers the problem I want to point out: the rash application of the language of imagery to an analytical framework that translates into an ethical act. Haraway and Agamben serve as a theoretical anchor for the demonization of organ transplants. Here, Haraway has been taken out of context: lacking the socialist–feminist program she seeks to further in "A Cyborg Manifesto," any use of her "Cyborg Manifesto" is only an empty frame. All Scheper-Hughes is seeking to do is to form an association between the cyber-organism image and the body image she associates with organ transplants. But without the ironic barb, on the one hand, and the political edge, on the other hand, that Haraway presented in her classic article, all that remains is the grotesque body image, a frozen analogy.

Then, Agamben appears: his model of "exposed life" is presented as it relates to life after transplantation. The trace of Faustianism sneaks in once again: the false promise of (mad?) science in league with economic interests. In the resultant atmosphere of decadence, this science offers "select individuals of reasonable economic means," a potion of youth that turns out to be more of a curse than a blessing. Agamben's notion of the bios relates to life bereft of humanness, a life of the body alone, which appears here as a description of life after transplantation. When the article appeared in 2000, such a description seemed somewhat strange, given the institutionalization of organ transplants as routine medicine as early as the 1980s. While the criticism of positivism does allow for the course carried out by Scheper-Hughes, nevertheless, the distance between Agamben's concept of the exposed life and a description of the lives of organ recipients is still great. Furthermore, such an analogy creates a misrepresentation of organ transplants; it flattens the complexity of the relationship between transplant medicine and processes of globalization to a spectacle of black against white.

Combining sensationalist language, the cyborg image, and the Faustian traces, Scheper-Hughes shows transplantation medicine in an absolutely grotesque light. In the article quoted here, as in a whole series of articles (one of the first of which [1998] was entitled "The New Cannibalism"), Scheper-Hughes sallies forth to document the global trade in human organs (Scheper-Hughes 2005, 2003, 2002, 1998). Her critical stance leads her to shatter the picture of the universe as we know it, which differentiates, among other things, between organ transplants and organ trafficking, and she sees in this medicine, in general, "a blend of altruism and commerce; of science and superstition; of gifting, barter, and theft; and of voluntarism and coercion...it has redefined real/unreal, seen/unseen, life/death, body/corpse/cadaver, person/nonperson, and rumor/fiction/fact" (Scheper-Hughes 2000:193). In this context, it is not at all clear to begin with what organ transplants are. Scheper-Hughes denies what she considers to be no more than an ideological cloak:

> Several key words in organ transplantation require radical deconstruction, among them "scarcity," "need," donation," "gift," bond," "life," "death," "supply," and "demand." Organ scarcity, for example, is invoked like a mantra in reference to the long waiting lists of candidates for various transplant surgeries....But this scarcity, created by the technocrats of transplant surgery, represents an artificial need, one that can never be satisfied, for underlying it is the unprecedented possibility of extending life indefinitely with the organs of others. I refer, with no disrespect intended to those now patiently waiting for organ transplants, to the age-old denial and refusal of death...Meanwhile, the so-called gift of life that is extended to terminal heart, lung, and liver patients is sometimes something other than the commonsense notion of a life. The survival rates of a great many transplant patients often conceal the real living-in-death—the weeks and months of extended suffering—that precedes actual death. Transplant patients today are increasingly warned that they are not exchanging a death sentence for a new life but rather exchanging one mortal, chronic disease for another
>
> (Scheper-Hughes 2000:198)

Scheper-Hughes' criticism seeks to expose the ideological cloak that conceals the hard truth about organ transplantation. But, what Scheper-Hughes does, in fact, is depicting transplant medicine in a series of dichotomies, where the utopian promise of a new medical technology is nothing but a dystopian nightmare of medicine gone wild. Thus, for her, the promise of life is the promise of death and shortage is surfeit. Following this line, the gift of life, thus, is the gift of death: not only do transplants make use of organs from deceased donors, but the very guarantee of life is a guarantee of suffering and agonized death. Not only that – at the place where we are accustomed to seeing a shortage, we are in fact seeing deception: "The real scarcity," writes Scheper-Hughes further on in the article, "is not of organs but of transplant patients of sufficient means to pay for them" (p. 199). Beyond the Orwellian sensation, this move by Scheper-Hughes actually sterilizes the criticism of its barb, since depicting the transplant medicine as a dystopia, making a sweeping condemnation of any and all organ transplants, undermines those trying to understand the nature of the problem of transplantation and the danger inherent in the organ trade without throwing out the baby with the bathwater.

The object of Scheper-Hughes' research project is the global trade in organs. Her method includes not only interviews and observations but also folk tales – myths, urban legends, and rumors culled from the ethnographic expeditions of Scheper-Hughes and her colleagues on three continents. The gathering of the data is not systematic, but documentation is problematic in any case in the underworld of organ trafficking. At the same time, basing knowledge about organ trafficking on oral rumors is no mere default in a field where there's more than meets the eye. The profusion of urban legends and folk myths about organ transplants is also instructive regarding the locals' resistance and mistrust of medicine, science, technology, and the western regime of knowledge, in general. Critical anthropology has taught us that the baseless rumor, the confused narrative, the myth, and the urban legend produce the alternative regime of knowledge of the subaltern, a field of knowledge juxtaposed with the western regime of knowledge, in general, and medicine, in particular. Folklore, rumor, and legend usurp the place of the factualism and positivism of medicine. In the research before us, the object of the research – transplant medicine – emerges as the loser. A reading of Scheper-Hughes' articles indicates that organ trafficking is an inevitable consequence of transplant medicine in a capitalist age. The boundaries between transplants and trafficking in organs are blurred in such writing, so much so that it is no longer clear whether the critics' arrows are aimed at the evils of organ trafficking, the practice of transplantation itself, or perhaps both.

The editors of *Current Anthropology*, in which the article appeared, presented eight responses by anthropologists from around the world, alongside the article together with images taken from Scheper-Hughes and her colleagues' field work.[2] Thus, a peek was offered into the evolution of ethnography regarding trade/transplantation of organs in the field of anthropological discourse:

> While reading this article I also happened to be reading Michael Taussig's *Shamanism, Colonialism, and the Wildman* and thought it only a coincidence, therefore, when these two seemingly unrelated works intersected. They intersected in the image—created by an early-20th-century missionary recording his encounter with savagery in the upper Amazon—of Indians playing a ball game with what they called the heart of Jesus. It was a ball made of rubber, the same commodity that was extracted through the atrocities of debt peonage, a commodity at the base of profound terror

[referring to colonialism—H.B.]—an organ transplant of a different sort. But is it so different?

(Alter 2000:222)

"The heart of Jesus," the rubber ball of Amazon natives, is the metaphor adopted by Taussig to indicate those natives' use of the metaphor (the heart of Jesus as a ball kicked over and over again) as allegory for missionary work and resistance, colonialism, and localism. But, Alter takes the allegory further and adds on another level, this time between "the heart of Jesus," with all its subversive, post-colonial connotations, and organ transplants. The second level of the allegory unravels the difference between organ trafficking and organ transplantation, since at this stage it is already difficult to distinguish between metaphors about the body and metaphors about exploitation, between the cultural meanings of organ transplants and the critical meanings opposing organ trade: "In the case of organ transplants there is something similar going on," Alter writes after another quotation from the rituals of the Amazon Indians,

> but the body takes on meaning and value not as a whole but only, or at least primarily, in terms of its various parts, producing a cannibalism that selectively nibbles—a gourmet cannibalism in which the "void erupting at the moment of a ritualized death" is also the "gift of life." In other words, I think transplant surgery fetishizes life to such an extent that it makes it possible to see the world, in a magically real sort of way, as populated by "immortal" body parts under the management of mortal souls. Cannibalism and capitalism are mutually constitutive by means of death and consumption, but transplant surgery and global neoliberal capitalism produce a moral space where life and death consume one another in a feast of difference that never ends.

> (ibid)

Evidently, it is Alter's argument that the combination of organ transplants with capitalism of necessity leads to organ trafficking. But, this claim is expressed in a way that does not differentiate between transplants and trade and offers no explanation or analysis, but only the play of images in which we quickly find ourselves discussing the mutual constitution of cannibalism and capitalism.

The thrust of Scheper-Hughes' discussion is the interrelationships of capitalism, globalization, commodification, and transplantation, but the discussion does not rise above organ trafficking as simply a further example of the evils of globalization. Marcelo Suárez-Orozco writes in response to Scheper-Hughes' article:

> Most postindustrial democracies have developed a voracious appetite for foreign bodies to do the impossible jobs that nobody wants to do....Today there are well over 100 million immigrants in the world...I sense that the movement of body parts and of immigrant workers is one-way: periphery to core, south to north, poor to rich.

> (Suárez-Orozco 2000:218)

Indeed, organ trafficking is an integral part of the systems of exploitation that have become more powerful by virtue of globalization's neo-liberalism. But, the truth must be told: the trade in organs for transplantation is limited and anecdotal in scope when compared with the global trade in human beings for purposes of sex and work. In relation to these trade cycles, the trade in organs is limited to a relatively small population of those in need of transplants.[3] The tendency to assign organ trafficking in the same line with all of globalization's political economic crimes does not result from its scope or even its grievousness[4] but from the way that rhetoric, in the semantic combining of "trade" or "trafficking" and "organs," affects our moral imagination. The collocation "organ trafficking" arouses our disgust as entailing all of the wickedness in the relationships of inequality among human beings. "Organ trafficking" is hyperbole, an indulgence that western culture can no longer afford to tolerate. In "organ trafficking," we see an exaggeration of the implications of inequality between people, an exaggeration of the concept of merchandise, and an exaggeration of the economic logic of capitalism. The expression, thus, serves as a receptacle for all the wrongs built into the very logic of capitalism, thereby creating a safety valve that permits the exploitation of labor by directing attention and the criticism of capitalism to the exploitation of body rather than the exploitation of labor.

In this way, organ trafficking has come to exemplify the decadence of the economic and technological order of the end of the millennium (Comaroff and Comaroff 1999). "Organ trafficking" is a dead metaphor; it no longer needs interpretation. Rather, it makes itself clear from the very semantic signification it contains: trading in organs. Trading in living human organs. There is no need for any further explanation, no need to draw a picture. The association gives rise to horror. Criticism is inherent in the very nature of the collocation "organ trafficking," a phrase that encompasses commodification, dissected body images, and the pernicious processes of unfettered medicalization. The next step is the moral one – a world populated by "surplus bodies," "strange markets," "Kula necklaces of human organs," similar to the end stages of what Oswald Spengler called "the decline of the West" (1932); the end of culture comes with the mastery of money and machine over the cycles of life. This is the essence of the world of organ trade, as presented to us by critical medical anthropologists.

In such a somber world, it is clear what side should be taken. In 1999, Scheper-Hughes founded an organization called "Organs Watch," which documented and reported on cases of organ trafficking. Her research served as the basis for her testimony before a special council of the US Senate, and in 2008, she participated in the World Health Organization's Declaration of Istanbul, which prohibited all forms of organ trading within and between nations. Scheper-Hughes deserves credit for her role in the war against organ trafficking, but, in fact, by referring to the trade in organs as an example of boundless commodification under the patronage of medicine, and in obscuring the difference between transplantation and trafficking, Scheper-Hughes forfeits her credibility in nuanced analysis in favor of moral denunciation. One image is worth a thousand words, and glib wording spares one the trouble of finding shades and nuances. The sweeping juxtaposition between transplantation medicine, capitalism, commodification, globalization, and body images leads to the assumption that organ trafficking is the expression of choice for the phenomenon of organ transplantation in the age of capitalism. But, beyond this general claim, it still is not clear what the institutional mechanisms that create various degrees of merchandising and privatization are, and whether there is any delineation between the various types of donation and commodification. Moreover, the blurring of the boundaries between trafficking and transplantation and the tendency to use body symbolism or the connection between capitalism, medicine, and ethics to study transplant medicine ultimately leads to the farfetched position that almost automatically casts doubt on the realia of transplantation.

In other words, the hermeneutics of suspicion realizes its aims in every facet of transplantation, thereby emptying not only the object of the criticism of all substance but also the effectiveness of the criticism itself. When the suspicion spills over in this research method, in a stroke of supreme irony it becomes a certainty regarding the unavoidable decadence of transplant medicine. Essential attributes of the universe of transplantation are denied in favor of moral condemnation. Thus, as noted above, the scarcity of organs for transplantation is described by Scheper-Hughes as "artificial needs and invented scarcities" (Scheper-Hughes 2000:198), and this note is also repeated by Cohen (2001) and to some degree also by Sharp (2006). The ability of organ transplantation to save lives and to dramatically enhance the quality of life of those needing dialysis is also at the very least repressed in this discourse, and organ transplantation is frequently referred to as a kind of experimental medicine which, while it may extend life, nevertheless destroys the humanness of the recipients and condemns them to a life in which, in the words of Alter quoted above, "'immortal' body parts [are] under the management of mortal souls." The temptation to use parallelism (immortal body parts – mortal souls) eclipses the fact that not only are transplanted organs not immortal, but the central challenge of transplantation is to slow the rate of their rejection, that is, their destruction by the recipient's natural immune system. When the moral condemnation is based on facile language, the grasp of the essential characteristics of the field of research vanishes in favor of an eddy of metaphors, and language is a casualty of language.

Although the tendency toward a "hermeneutic of suspicion" is engraved on the critical position, still this position often leads to misgivings as to the fundamental components of the political economy of organ transplants. Not only is the challenge of acceptance and rejection of the implant – the very essence of transplantation – disconnected from its material foundation in favor of symbolic representation. The scarcity of organs and the degree of success in organ transplantation are also seen as random, as being dependent on one's point of view. In fact, it is the problem of scarcity and the medical successes of organ transplantation that are the central factors making organ trafficking possible. The erasure and obscuring of the boundaries between trafficking in and transplanting organs cause a simplistic view of a world of good versus bad, the innocent versus the villains, authentic culture versus corruptive technology, and we are left without a more comprehensive systemic explanation of the phenomenon. Instead of a general explanation, critical medical anthropology offers us a discussion that constantly veers between a poetic representation of images of the transplanted body and moral condemnation of the ethical order for which an image of the transplanted body is nothing but its metonymy.

Laurence Cohen, in his research on the organ trade in India in the late 1990s, addresses the pharmacological developments that led to improved acceptance of the transplanted organ and made the matching process simpler. These developments – the creation of a pharmaceutical cocktail to suppress the recipient's immune system – have expanded the population of potential candidates for organ donation. For Cohen, this cocktail also possesses characteristics of social subjection:

> Despite the promise of immune recognition and tissue-typing for the rise of an effective transplant medicine, it was not the recognition of molecular sameness and difference but the *suppression* [italics in the original] of the entire system of code that ultimately materialized the population—rather, specific populations—as viable donors. Suppression, not recognition, turned transplantation into a major industry.
>
> (Cohen 2001:11)

Indeed, the marketing of immunosuppressant drugs has transformed transplant medicine into a global success story. Today, when we are already in the third generation of immunosuppressant drugs, the challenge is not a perfect match but actually the lack of a match: transplantation is a viable option even without a perfect match. It should be borne in mind that pharmacological developments have not yet resolved the issue of rejection; a transplanted organ is destined for rejection. All that can be done is to slow the rate of rejection of the organ. Today, recipients can live long lives, rather than the few years that was common in the 1970s. But, the appearance of the first immunosuppressant drug already worried Cohen, since expanding the population of candidates for organ donation meant more possibilities for exploitation. This is precisely what happened when India expanded its population of donor candidates. Cohen claims that the transplant medical teams are not interested in immunological sameness or physiological profile, but in the eradication of this sameness so that the transplantation might succeed. However, I wish to point out that exploitation is caused not by technology but by its combination with a socioeconomic structure. The parasite of technological exploitation leads first to adoption of a position of "technological determinism," next to the ineradicable assertion that organ transplantation is a technology of exploitation, and finally, to an intensification of the horror aroused by organ transplantation. This discursive orientation of Cohen's further obscures the difference between transplantation and organ trafficking and strengthens the criticism and demonization of any and all organ transplants:

> Just when we thought that the metonymic late modern life science was immunology, *surgery*—that hoary cynosure of an early modern medicine—emerges to

reclaim the field. The endless cybernetic narrative of medical management—adjusting inputs and outputs to accommodate failing organs at the level of the total system—is replaced by the possibility of a continual circulation of spare parts….Under the sign of the transplant [surgery itself] may be shifting….we are becoming bags of organs. If one of the contents of the bag (or the bag itself) is damaged or wears out, we can now imagine a sequence of continual replacement…Life, for those who are able to occupy the position of such a patient, promises a future of a stutter between surgeries.

(Cohen 2001:23)

The confusion between trafficking and transplantation of organs is understandable if one considers the socioeconomic context of organ transplants in India. But, here, the criticism goes far beyond this: like Scheper-Hughes and Alter, cited above, Cohen exaggerates the advantage enjoyed by organ transplantation (is the situation really one of "continual replacement"?) over the image ("bags of organs"). The interweaving of the image within the exaggeration about the power of transplant surgery, about the impact of the immunosuppressant drugs or the action of the immune system places us again in a Faustian universe in which medicine, as Illich (1976) says, does more harm than good.

The temptation to resort to such transplantation concepts as suppressants of the immune system as a metaphor for the social face of this medicine is also clearly seen in Joralemon's ethnography. For Joralemon, the challenge in the suppression of the immune system to allow the body to accept the implant parallels the challenge in the suppression of the cultural system to facilitate the acceptance of transplantation as conventional medicine. "What I am arguing is that, at least for the present and near future, the cultural success of transplantation will be measured by how effectively its supporting ideology suppresses, rather than replaces, traditional concepts of bodily integrity" (Joralemon 1995:347). This, however, is myopic. The viability of organ transplants depends on a much more complex array of delays and obstructions: beyond the distrust and opposition noted by Joralemon, successful recruitment of organs for transplantation depends on far more prosaic factors, such as the logistical coordination between hospitals, the establishment of an apparatus of transplant coordinators, standardization of tissue typing, an expeditious system of ensuring compatibility between donor and patient, and so on (Machado 1998, Hogle 1995).

The critical anthropology's perspective on organ transplants is interesting because it teaches us a great deal about methodological symbolism and critical investigation about the danger in conflating research and moral judgment. Apparently, in the case of organ transplantation, the irresistibility of metaphorical language has reached its peak. The discourse is usually bifurcated. First, an image is created to describe the practice itself, at which point the image becomes a metaphor; that is, the qualities of the image point to the qualities in a different field of meaning. The second step is the transformation of the metaphor into an allegory about the social order so that finally the denunciation and censure become clear. The founding text of Swazey and Fox in transplantation anthropology illustrates the process clearly. The expression "spare parts" to describe organ transplants was chosen by Swazey and Fox as the title of their book, and in the short quotation introduced at the beginning of this sub-section, at least three images appear: the authors recoil from a universe of "man-machine unions," of "rebuilt people," and of "prosthetized humans." All of these lead Swazey and Fox to abandon the universe of transplantation, not because of exhaustion and burnout but of a growing alarm as to the future. Actually, these authors are recoiling from the universe of images they themselves created. The recoiling results from the persuasive power of the image, and all their writing is nothing but a stage in the mythologizing of organ transplantation.

Utopia – the gift of life discourse

In an opposite mirror reflection of the dystopian discourse of critical medical anthropology is the transplantation and organ donation glorifying discourse that can be termed as "the gift of life" discourse. This discourse is carried out by a gamut of agents: health professionals, ad agencies, media advisors, and public relations experts hired by official health authorities to promote awareness to organ donation and signing donor cards. Health experts, especially transplantation personnel, are also part of the construction of the image of the benefactor in transplantation. They often speak in the name of science and claim a central position in bioethical debates on transplantation and are in constant confrontation with medical anthropology's critical discourse. One of the first public figures who directly confronted the hermeneutics of suspicion discourse was Jean Hamburger, who performed the first kidney transplant in 1952 in France. In 1979, he published a book that could be considered a rejoinder to the criticism of medicalization, in general, and of dialysis and kidney transplantation, in particular. The book, *Demain, les autres*, tells the story of the artificial kidney (dialysis) and of kidney transplants as a story of promise, of hope for the future. The original French title, Tomorrow: the Others, is germane to our discussion. Its concern is twofold: the future (tomorrow) and the fate that this future bears for the social fabric (others). The combination of the two produces the hermeneutics of hope, the designation of the horizon as being better, and technology and science as the vehicle to take us into this future. In contrast to Swazey and Fox's *The Courage to Fail* and Ivan Illich's *Medical Nemesis*, which were published several years before, Hamburger, discussing dialysis and the early kidney transplantations, does not see any tension between the social and the medical. For him, technological developments cannot realize their full potential without the cooperation of the community (Hamburger 1979).[5]

Hamburger published his book a few years before the pharmacological revolution broke in the early 1980s. This revolution ushered in effective medications for the suppression of the immune system without causing serious and immediate damage to the other systems of the body and in so doing transformed transplantation into a routine medical procedure. Dated to the eve of this revolution, Hamburger's book provides interesting testimony from the establishment point of view, since it was written during the experimental period of transplantation, when not infrequently transplant operations ended in failure and when the survival rate of the recipients was much shorter than today.[6] Yet, Hamburger's book describes the evolution of transplantation medicine and dialysis treatments in heroic terms. Rationally debating the critics, Hamburger polemicizes against the heart of the critical claim about medicalization and medical hubris. He describes the pioneering experiments in the construction of the dialysis machine and his first collaboration as a nephrologist in the 1950s and 1960s with Belding Scribner, a colleague from the United States, who devised the idea of dialysis. Hamburger describes the tension between science, medicine, and ethics.

> In the course of my conversation with Belding Scribner before he set about testing his bold idea, my only questions had to do with nephrology. But in my heart of hearts I pondered: the problem was not limited to technical obstacles. It was hard to believe a person would be willing to spend so many hours in a hospital, connected to a machine, two or three times a week—until the end of his life! How could a person bear the idea of being so dependent, with the sword of death waving over his head should he take even a short break from his treatments? Even if it were only a matter of being connected to an artificial kidney for a few days—in a case of severe uremia—great pains must sometimes be taken to keep the patient from despairing. What would happen, then, in a treatment that must last all one's life? But I was very wrong. And I want to learn the lessons of my mistake.
>
> (Hamburger 1979:114)

The idea of life in the age of technology is presented here in all its acuteness. The technology exists, but the cost seems too great: a life of unremitting suffering, too hard to bear. At this point, Hamburger's claim is similar to the one we encountered above regarding exposed life, a life of suffering under the burden of medical technology. But, Hamburger immediately proceeds to unload this tension in the opposite direction, producing an interpretive rejoinder antithetical to what we have seen in the mechanism of the discourse of suspicion:

> The latest statistics show that over half the patients needing periodic hemodialysis are potential candidates (from the standpoint of their age, the state of their health, and their qualifications) for full-time work (...) A certain music critic never worked as prolifically as after he started treatment. There's an artist with a similar story. A certain statesman resumed his diplomatic activity with renewed enthusiasm, where until his dialysis it had looked as though he would have to forsake it forever. A woman who until then had no success in her emotional life and had almost despaired of trying her luck again is now making a new life for herself. But these wonderful changes and manifestations of courage are only part of the story. They certainly testify to the daring that some men and women are capable of, and they are a response, a kind of cry of defiance against a fate of suffering and grievance. I need to

describe the saga of hundreds and thousands of anonymous patients who are simply and modestly taking up their lives again in spite of their suffering. Mute valor. Or, if you prefer, life, a hard life that goes on, and as hard as it is, so much better than the grave (…) One who is forced to use an artificial kidney is unquestionably unfortunate, or should I say fortunate? (…) There have been those who found God when times were hard, who had never been close to Him before. Others only found life—a life filled with horrible events but also with the wonders of every day.

(Hamburger 1979:114)

The concept of life itself is put to the test here. How are we to understand life in the age of medical technology? This question may be translated into one regarding the benefit of transplantation, or in the above passage, of dialysis treatments. But, the question of benefit is but one dimension of a larger question regarding the condition of life itself in the age of medical technology. From this standpoint, organ transplantations and dialysis treatments constitute a private matter for discussion of the implications of processes of medicalization or of medicine's encroachment on how the concept of life in modern society is molded. And from this standpoint, Hamburger's writing is critical to an understanding of the positive point of view and its justifications in a time of experimental transplantation medicine. Interestingly, his point of departure does not nullify the suspicions that the value of life in the technological era will erode: in the first passage, he acknowledges that he shuddered to contemplate living with dialysis for a long time. Neither does he belittle the magnitude of the suffering these treatments involve later in the paragraph. His argument infuses an interpretation that pays tribute to the dialysis treatments and the patients "who are simply and modestly taking up their lives again in spite of their suffering."

This is an uncommon attitude regarding the tension between suffering and hope, and it is hard to find more attitudes like it in the establishment discourse about organ transplantations. In fact, the formal ethical view sees the living conditions under dialysis as a sufficiently viable alternative to the ethical problems they see in kidney transplantation, and the "fate of suffering and grievance," in the words of Hamburger, pales when compared to a purpose unsullied by hardship and suffering. While in the early years of transplantation and the technology of the artificial kidney, the dimension of suffering was presented as the price of trailblazing in medicine, since the early 1980s the hermeneutics of hope has framed the dramas of courage played out in transplantation in visual images in which the dangers, the hardships, the fact that "people must die," as the ethicist Youngner (2003) puts it, translate into body images of the I/other combined within the recipient's body and bestow life to the one and consolation to the other.

"The gift of life," metaphor has become the leading image in this glorifying discourse. The image has undergone an intensive process of branding and marketing by donation encouragement public campaigns so that it is read as literally the actual giving of life. Actually, it hides the political economy of such gifts and the social conditions that determine the donation, rendering the act as an act of pure grace and deed. While I am not doubting at all the pure motivations that often lead to organ donations, the concept of the gift has more anthropological bearings than meets the eye. The "gift of life" idiom camouflages the complex relationship between giver and receiver to the point that there are cases in which the gift of life has been transformed into "a fallacy" (Siminoff and Chillag 1999). Siminoff and Chilag have noticed that in promoting the gift of life paradigm, the recipients are expected to express even greater compliance to their post-operative regime since their enhanced feelings of indebtedness. This, indeed, can be a source of mental strain for the indebtedness organ recipient who could never return an equivalent to her savior.

The metaphor conceals reality and presents an image. The "gift of life" metaphor transfers the complex reality of the one person giving an organ to another to the universe of images of unconditional giving, of the ultimate giving a human can provide, which is next to a divine ability: giving life. Organ donation does have dimensions of unconditional giving, of "a gift" to a certain degree, but it is a giving that exists in the context of discernible social institutions: does the donation of an organ within the family qualify as having the same gift-like characteristics as the anonymous organ donation from a corpse? Or in other cases, taking an organ from someone under the assumption that anyone would agree to such a "gift" unless he declares otherwise, as in the presumed consent system of organ procurement?

Clearly, the "gift of life" transfers a variety of practices of organ donation to a different register, largely analogized to limitless generosity. Furthermore, the "gift of life" image endows the giver with a feeling of transcendence, thus taking its place beside a succession of Promethean images of transplantation medicine. While it is true that every medical intervention is to one degree or another an intervention in creation, the "gift of life" image positions us in an area in which it is not the doctors who bestow life through their art and the tools at their disposal, but rather the individual who chooses to cooperate with the medical system. Prometheus is not the doctor intervening in an area reserved for God and nature, but rather the individual, any individual, choosing to donate organs.

"The gift of life" image is tempting, because it colors the practice of transplantation in a way that severs it, so to speak, from the cultural context of barter in the modern world. Just as the expression "organ trafficking" jolts us from the juxtaposition of the words "trafficking" and "organs," so too does the expression "the gift of life" not leave us unaffected. The very juxtaposition of the words "gift" and "life" transports us to lofty spheres. In both linguistic instances, we actually find ourselves at the junction between economics and morality, except that whereas the expression "organ trafficking" reduces transplantation medicine to the level of decadent technology and capitalism run rampant, the expression "gift of life" elevates it to a level of heightened morality.

This is exactly the see-saw of images in which the discourse about transplantation takes place. Actually, "gift of life" and "organ trafficking" resonate off each other: each is formulated in each of the mechanisms of discourse as silencing and denial of the opposing expression. In point of fact, organ trade gives life, and also in the gift of life, there is an active and clear discourse of barter; the "gift of life" is undeniably a budget item in hospital, Health Ministry, and welfare office account books. In neither expression is there a clear demarcation between these two discursive fields; they are intertwined in a sort of a mebius ring of morality so that it is unclear when moral categories are exogenous or indigenous.

The positive view of the gift of life is also expressed in an optimism and trust in medical technology. Against the decadent image enveloping transplantation medicine in the discourse of critical medical anthropology, in the optimistic take on organ transplantations, we find reversed working assumptions that produce an image of technological progress which opens the door not only to the great breakthrough in medical history but also to new forms of communal ties, social cohesion, collective solidarity, and altruism. These presumptions feature the mainstream discourse on transplant medicine, promoted mainly by official health agencies. The role of metaphors, images, and idioms is central in this discourse as well. Similar to the critical discourse on transplantations, we also find here images of a modular, rebuilt body, selfhood and otherness, and technology and society. In the mainstream discourse, however, these metaphors serve to depict transplant medicine as a utopia of moral, technological, biomedical, and social progress. Transplantation medicine is conceived as the sublime apex of modernism, the meeting point not just of organs from different bodies but also the trajectories of a social morality and bio-technological developments. In the making of organ transplantations as a utopia, as well as in its reversed parallel, the language of metaphors and images produces ideological screens that renders transplantation medicine pure white or evil black.

Transplant medicine is depicted as reaching scientific and moral peak at once: a donor's organs are allocated to dying patients: one heart, two kidneys, liver lobes, lungs, and pancreas are only the solid organs that can save the life of up to eight dying patients, not to mention tissues, such as corneas. The division between the body and its parts, the dead body and its living parts, is depicted as a moral horizon in the landscape of our materialistic society. Campaigns for increasing public awareness to transplantations render this aspect a central axis of metaphor. Thus, for instance, the story of Yael Alony and Omri Gilor, whose heart was transplanted in her body in 2008, is introduced in an official clip of the Israeli Transplant Center, as the story of the self and the other intertwined in one body. With a violin playing in the background, we see Yael dancing together with friends in a ballet class, laughing and having fun with friends and family, jumping to the swimming pool, and hugging with her sister and brother. A baritone voice over reads: "Her look is her mother's look, her talents is her grandmother's talent, her laugh is her grandfather's laugh, her courage is certainly from her mother". And then, the music stops and we hear heartbeats. The camera passes from her smiling face to her scarred chest and then the interlocutor says: "and her heart, her healthy heart, Yael received from Omri, whose family consented to organ donation."

This strong clip identifies genetic heritance with organ donation; a close warming imaging of organ donors as family members. The heart was chosen by no accidence, the heart is the most metaphoric organ of all. It corresponds with giving, love, devotion, to the inner self. The overall feeling is of a warm embracing family, of organ donation as a re-birth. In 2011, Yael was 12, the exact age in which Omri died. His heart still kept her alive.

The image of a transplanted heart is a central and strong image in the utopic and the dystopic depictions of organ transplantations. In a reversed constellation of images and contexts that Alter found in the Amazonian "Jesus heart" play, Omri's heart becomes a synecdoche for giving, love, and intimacy. "I cannot understand how one cannot consent to organ donation" wrote one person as a feedback to the internet story of Yael and Omri. Images of human bodies integrated in each other introducing the message that we are all but one human tissue are the symbols of transplant organizations worldwide. "Don't take your heart to heaven, heaven knows we need it here" is another organ donation famous slogan. The image of the transplanted body invites us to the world where consenting to donation is parallel to the blessing of giving life. This is solicitation via utopian description which renders the donor a miracle-maker, a God.

In fact, perhaps the most central idiom in the mainstream discourse of organ transplantation is the "Gift of Life." Organ donation as the gift of life became such a pervasive idiom so that it appears not just in the PR imaging of organ transplantation but also in legal acts such as the US Uniform Anatomical Gift Act. But, the gift of life is not just a buzz word, it is the metonym of the utopian understanding of organ transplant such as "organ trafficking" is the synecdoche of its dystopia, both metaphors operate in the sphere of economy and morality. Both mark the ending points of a moral economy. Both need not further explanations. They are self-evident, empty metaphors. The gift of life emphasizes the voluntarily act of giving as an act of a God-like grace. The donor is apotheosized and aggrandized as having the ability to grant life. In the gift of life, we meet organ donation as an omnipotent act. This miraculous status becomes with transplant medicine, an item of choice in modern life's menu. Each one of us, by consenting to organ donation, whether in her life time, after death and in consenting to donate your loved one's organs, can transcend to the level of God-giving-life. According to the intensive donor cards campaign, it is enough to declare on a future, nonbinding, consent and to sign on donor card in order to win the potential of being an altruist.

So, intensive is the institutionalization of the "gift of life" so that it is easy to forget that it is basically an idiom, a metaphor. The anthropology of gifts reminds us that gifts are always embed in an exchange economy. In fact, anthropological accounts have placed the gift as propelling social structuring. In gifts economy, there is a tradeoff between giver and taker and clear conditions of how to give and how to return gifts. A more detailed account on how transplantation medicine adopted the anthropology of the gift will be introduced in Chapter 4, it is sufficed, at this stage, to say that gifts are far from a one-sided, altruistic behavior. Its key function is to transport the reality of organ exchange to the imagined sphere of utopia.

Toward new anthropology of organ transplantations

At least four fundamental questions of anthropology are inherent in organ transplantation: the configuration of nature versus culture, the relationship between the self and the other, the definitions of life and death, and the social significance of the body. Thus, organ transplantations are transformed into an instrument to facilitate thinking about culture. They hardly remain within the bounds of medical protocol and rather go far beyond to the realm where they are transformed to metaphors and allegories. Transplantations have been presented through appearances as the grotesque body as an example of the all-encompassing manner in which processes of medicalization disrupt the order of the world or as the emblem of altruism. As image, as text, as allegory, organ transplants are often presented solely in connection with their metaphorical mantle. Thus, the language of metaphor continues to hold organ transplants in captivity of binary imagination that tilts between the sublime and the decadent.

For me, delving into the anthropological discourse on transplantations was a real shock. Unlike Fox and Swazey, I – like other organ recipients, patients on the waiting lists, or even the donors/sellers – will be forever bounded to this world and its ethical dilemmas. The privilege of Swazey and Fox in deciding to simply leave the field creates a rift between the researchers and their field. When deciding to write on organ transplant, I found myself specifically on the suture between the two roles: a researcher and a patient. Both discourses – the dystopic and utopic – seem to me, from my standpoint, to be serving other purposes, external to the distressing experience of waiting for an organ. Together, the utopic and dystopic narrative formed this moebius ring of morality where I felt lost. I had to come up with a new way to think about transplant medicine.

Against these discourses, this book offers an alternative method of analysis. Although it is almost impossible to free from the language of metaphors and adapt a free-images language (Lakoff and Jhonson 1980),[7] I suggest in the following chapters to study transplantations by reversing the analysis direction – instead of thinking about the morals of organ transplantations – utopian or dystopian – I wish to focus on organs themselves, and understand ethics and morality as emergent properties that are dependent on the different routes that organs take in their journey from one body to another. In this way, the in-between moral space – this which is neither sublime nor decadent – will be exposed in a more nuanced analysis. Specifically, instead of moral economy, the following chapters unfold a story of political economy, an economy of organs for transplantations.

In this way, it is first possible to move away from the methodological symbolism that dominated the current discourse – both utopian and dystopian – and second, shy away from imported concepts and ready-made categories, and understand the materialistic groundings that render ethical concepts and moral judgments their legitimacy and discursive volume. In a sense, I adapt a nominalistic approach, which is both realistic and yet rich enough to capture cultural constructs.

I do not wish to camouflage the moral dilemmas of organ transplantations or quickly present them only to purify them with a triumphant moral economy; it is out of the paradox – of that mebius ring – that locks moral judgment in a black and white opposing images that the research on transplant medicine can begin. In this respect, an anthropology of transplantations should begin by shunning away from normative or critical premises about the link between transplantations and morality, not because the conflicting moral economies of transplant medicine are incorrect but because it is exactly this link that should be under investigation. Adopting a moral economy as the normative framework might blind from observing the crowded paradoxes and hybrids that populate this world.

I suggest investigating into the world of transplant medicine by focusing on the core of the paradoxical nexus between the natural and the cultural. The paradoxes of the transplanted organ as the double metonym of the saving and the degradation of life render the organ itself the methodological and theoretical starting point for deciphering the social universe of organ transplantations. The removed, transferred, circulated, transplanted, and sadly often rejected organ is the fundamental actor of this world; it is the quintessential mixture of nature and culture, the bearer of objectification and subjectification processes in a peculiar variant of political economy, it is both the hope and the despair of this world. In its course from the supplier to the recipient, the organ crosses different worlds of meanings and various moral regimes. Understanding the world of organ transplantation is to focus on the associations that bind the organ to different worlds and structure it in different moral, political, and economic constellations. The following chapters explore this method in unfolding the distinctive features of organ economy.

Notes

1 http://optn.transplant.hrsa.gov.
2 Most of the responses are positive with few reservations as to the methodology that Scheper-Hughes employed in her research.
3 While it is true that this population keeps on growing primarily due to the epidemics of diabetes and hypertension, organ transplantation is not first-line treatment, because of the high cost and scarcity of organs. See more on Chapter 4.
4 One can argue that organ trafficking has different levels of exploitation, deceit, and coercion. In black markets of organ trafficking, where the market is run by mafia or authoritative regime like in China, the coercion is graver and the risks for both buyer and seller are more concrete. In grey markets, there is more protection for the health of both parties. The lines, however, between black and grey markets are not fixed and a grey market can turn black. This is not to say that organ trafficking is legitimate or that even a regulated market is a good option. My normative stance is that organ trafficking is, indeed, an extreme case of privatization process (see Chapters 4 and 5) that was totally misrepresented by the anthropological discourse.
5 The following citations from this book were translated from its Hebrew version.
6 And its positive tone can be compared to critical voice of Fox and Swazey whose "Courage to Fail" published in 1974 and also refers to the experimental stage of pre-revolution of immunosuppressant agents.
7 See Lakoff and Jhonson (1980).

References

Alter, J. S. (2000) In response to Scheper-Hughes. *Current Anthropology*, 41(2), 222.

Bergan, A. (1997). Ancient myth, modern reality: A brief history of transplantation. *The Journal of Biocommunication*, 24(4), 2–9.

Cassell, E. J. (1993). The sorcerer's broom. *Hastings Center Report*, 23(6), 32–39.

Cohen, L. (2001). The other kidney: Biopolitics beyond recognition. *Body & Society*, 7(-2–3), 9–29.

Comaroff, J., & Comaroff, J. L. (1999). Occult economies and the violence of abstraction: Notes from the South African postcolony. *American Ethnologist*, 26(2), 279–303.

DiGiacomo, S. M. (1992). Metaphor as illness: Postmodern dilemmas in the representation of body, mind and disorder. *Medical Anthropology*, 14(1), 109–137.

Ellul, J. (1990). *The Technological Bluff*, MI: Eerdmans Grand Rapids.

Fox, R. C., & Swazey, J. P. (1992). *Spare Parts: Organ Replacement in American Society*, Oxford University Press.

Fox, R. C., & Swazey, J. P. (1974). *The Courage to Fail: A Social View of Organ Transplants and Dialysis*, Piscataway, NJ: Transaction Publications.

Gill, P., & Lowes, L. (2008). Gift exchange and organ donation: Donor and recipient experiences of live related kidney transplantation. *International Journal of Nursing Studies*, 45(11), 1607–1617.

Hamburger, J. (1979). *Demain, les autres: l'aventure medicale en contrepoint de l'aventure humaine*. Paris: Flammarion.

Helman, C. (1988). Dr. Frankenstein and the industrial body, *Anthropology Today*, 4(3), 14–16.

Hogle, L. F. (1995). Standardization across non-standard domains: The case of organ procurement. *Science, Technology & Human Values*, 20(4), 482–500.

Illich, I. (1976). *Limits to Medicine*, Marion Boyars.

Jonas, H. (1974). *Philosophical Essays: From Ancient Creed to Technological Man*, Englewood Cliffs, NJ: Prentice-Hall.

Jonas, H. (1969). Philosophical reflections on experimenting with human subjects. *Daedalus*, 98(2), 219–247.

Joralemon, D. (1995). Organ wars: The battle for body parts. *Medical Anthropology Quarterly*, 9(3), 335–356.

Kleinman, A. (1995). *Writing at the Margin: Discourse between Anthropology and Medicine*, Oakland, CA: University of California Press.

Lakoff, G., & Jhonson, M. (1980). *Metaphors We Live By*, Chicago: University of Chicago Press.

Machado, N. (1998). *Using the Bodies of the Dead: Legal, Ethical and Organizational Dimensions of Organ Transplantation*, London and New York: Routledge.

Morris, P. J. (2004). Transplantation—A medical miracle of the 20th century. *New England Journal of Medicine*, 351(26), 2678–2680.

Postman, N. (2011). *Technopoly: The Surrender of Culture to Technology*, Random House LLC.

Sanner, M. A. (2001). Exchanging spare parts or becoming a new person? People's attitudes toward receiving and donating organs. *Social Science & Medicine*, 52(10), 1491–1499.

Scheper-Hughes, N. (2005). The last commodity: Post-human ethics and the global traffic in "Fresh" organs. In Ong, A & Collier S.J. (eds). *Global Assemblages: Politics, and Ethics as Anthropological Problems*, Oxford: Blackwell Publishing. 145–167.

Scheper-Hughes, N. (2003). Rotten trade: Millennial capitalism, human values and global justice in organs trafficking. *Journal of Human Rights*, 2(2), 197–226.

Scheper-Hughes, N. (2002). Bodies for sale: whole or in parts. *Body & Society*, 7(2-3), 1–8.

Scheper-Hughes, N. (2001). Commodity fetishism in organs trafficking. *Body & Society*, 7(2–3), 31–62.

Scheper-Hughes, N. (2000). The global traffic in human organs. *Current Anthropology*, 41(2), 191–224.

Scheper-Hughes, N. (1998). The new cannibalism. *New Internationalist*, 300, 14–17.

Scheper-Hughes, N., & Lock, M. M. (1987). The mindful body: A prolegomenon to future work in medical anthropology. *Medical Anthropology Quarterly*, 1(1), 6–41.

Scheper-Hughes, N., & Lock, M. M. (1986). Speaking "Truth" to illness: Metaphors, reification, and a pedagogy for patients. *Medical Anthropology Quarterly*, 17(5), 137–140.

Scheper-Hughes, N., & Wacquant, L. (eds.). (2002). Commodifying bodies. *Body and Society*, 7(2–3). SAGE.

Sharp, L. A. (2006). *Strange Harvest: Organ Transplants, Denatured Bodies, and the Transformed Self*, Oakland, CA: University of California Press.

Sharp, L. A. (2001). Commodified kin: Death, mourning, and competing claims on the bodies of organ donors in the United States. *American Anthropologist*, 103(1), 112–133.

Sharp, L. A. (2000). The commodification of the body and its parts. *Annual Review of Anthropology*, 287–328.

Sharp, L. A. (1995). Organ transplantation as a transformative experience: Anthropological insights into the restructuring of the self. *Medical Anthropology Quarterly*, 9(3), 357–389.

Siminoff, L. A., & Chillag, K. (1999). The fallacy of the "gift of life". *Hastings Center Report*, 29(6), 34–41.

Sontag, S. (1977) *Illness as Metaphor*, New York: Farrar, Straus and Giroux.

Spengler, O. (1991) [1932]. *The Decline of the West*, Oxford University Press.

Suárez-Orozco, M. (2000) In response to Scheper-Hughes. *Current Anthropology*, 41(2), 218.

Tilney, N. L. (2003). *Transplant: From Myth to Reality*, New Haven, CT: Yale University Press.

Youngner, S. J. (2003). Some must die. *Zygon* 38(3), 705–724.

Tel Aviv 1999

It had been 13 years since my first transplant. It was an age of innocence: I lived under the impression that my nephrological problems had largely been solved by the transplant and that apart from periodic checkups, I could live a normal lifestyle. It wasn't a fanciful thought. In the 1980s and 1990s, transplantation medicine was developing rapidly and postoperative treatment based on suppressing the immune system significantly improved with the introduction of second- and third-generation immunosuppressive agents. Thus, I went through all of my high-school years trying to keep the story of my transplant and my life as a kidney transplantee out of view, as part of my private life. It was not a secret, but not something I immediately disclosed about myself either. My circle of close friends knew, and whoever didn't know eventually heard about it, or maybe not.

Looking back on those teenage years, I don't know if that way of presenting myself was correct. On the one hand, I was not like everyone else and I had restrictions. On the other hand, I went to a very competitive school and no digression from normality was welcome. The prevailing ethos was what current disability studies call the superman model: the disabled person overcomes their disability by themselves and succeeds despite it all to act by the norms of abled society. This superman concept, or disability as the possibility of heroism, is very problematic. It not only puts the burden of proving their heroism on the disabled person themselves but also fails to provide space for the disabled person's physical and emotional needs. But that was the dominant approach when I was an adolescent in the late 1980s and early 1990s, and only when I became a senior in high school, after years of receiving failing grades in sports, and in the year the boys began training for combat service (yes, my high school was also characterized by dated gender divisions), did I ask for and receive an exemption from those arduous phys. ed. classes.

Due to my medical condition, I was exempted from military service. But at that time I was determined to prove my normalcy, and I volunteered for military service and managed to pass the selection process for the military radio station. That is actually where I got to know the academic world. I served in the documentary contents department and edited and wrote short news flashes about scientific innovations. The service was a kind of correction to the depressing intellectual life of the high school, where only the natural sciences were considered serious

DOI: 10.4324/9781003288886-4

subjects. That was where I contracted the radio bug, which stayed with me for many years thereafter, mainly as a content editor who wished to bridge between the academia and the general public.

After my service, I had an overwhelming desire to study history. I signed up for a degree in history, and since a double major was required, I also signed up for the department of sociology and anthropology, mainly because Maya, my girlfriend at the time and my wife today, had signed up for it, and I wanted to study with her. I was fascinated by the university: I thought that for every word the lecturers uttered, they must have read a hundred. I thought they were the smartest people I had ever met. When I finished my bachelor's degree at the age of 24, I was offered to continue to a master's degree in sociology and to be a teaching assistant for introductory courses. It was an offer I could not refuse, even if it meant continuing in sociology rather than in history, which I preferred.

During my master's degree, I got to know academic life better. I was a TA, I taught and did research. I wrote a master's thesis about the political culture of secular–religious relations from the perspective of sociological history, published two articles, and was even invited to present one of them at a conference at Toronto University in Canada. At the end of my degree, a classmate told me the "facts of life" of academe in Israel. "If you want to have an academic career" – he told me what would, indeed, turn out to be one of the unwritten rules for those running the academic course – "you have to do a PhD abroad, preferably in the US." We signed up together in the summer for a preparatory course for the GREs, I asked my master's thesis supervisors for recommendation letters, and I applied to leading US universities.

A first crack in the emerging picture of academic studies came from a seemingly prosaic matter: health insurance. It is customary to apply for scholarships to fund graduate studies. I went to the Fulbright foundation, and in the preliminary requirements for the application, they required a sound health status that allows health insurance. I was particularly offended by that demand, considering the section that also asked for the specification of my contribution to the community. "This time I am asking you to contribute to the community," I wrote in my reply letter.

> My health does not meet the standard of a healthy person, and it is I who need your support in order to advance my plans to study in the US. Could you please pay for private health insurance for me?

I received a standard negative response with no reference to my special request.

It was especially unfortunate because I had already received positive answers from Northwestern University in Chicago and the University of San Diego in California (UCSD). That was, as I said, an age of innocence, and I believed I could find medical insurance on my own. What troubled me the most was going with Maya, my girlfriend at the time, to live in a distant and foreign place, a life designed mainly around my academic studies. Would our relationship survive it? Were we even cut out for living in the United States? Naïve as I was, I thought maybe we should go see the places where I was accepted, and then maybe we would be able to make a decision one way or another. After all, my relationship was more important to me than my PhD.

We planned the trip for September 1999. We thought we should go two or three weeks before the academic year began. Two days before the trip, I had an appointment for my periodic checkup at the hospital. Those days I used to do blood tests every three or six months, and my situation was relatively stable and did not concern me at all. That's why I was so shocked when the nephrologist looked at the test results and said: "You're not going anywhere, you're getting hospitalized immediately and starting dialysis."

I burst out crying. I couldn't help it. I had to call Maya and give her the bad news. I remember the call from the hospital payphone as if it were just yesterday. All of our plans were canceled: thoughts of the PhD in the United States, the trip in two days, and besides, whoever thought that the kidney could be rejected? In fact, only then did I realize that the life of a transplanted kidney is limited and it will ultimately be rejected. What would have happened had I been aware all those years of the fact of rejection and lived under that Sword of Damocles?

The reasons for rejection are not clear. The medical term is "chronic rejection" and it refers to a series of processes and reasons for which the transplanted kidney functions less and less effectively until the transplantee reaches a state of kidney failure that requires dialysis or transplantation. Why did I reject the kidney I had received from my father? I was very careful to take the pills and follow the medical instructions and directives, and my shock over the rejection of the kidney was absolute. The doctors offered a different point of view. As far as they were concerned, 13 years, from the transplant in 1986 to its rejection in 1999, were nothing less than an achievement to be proud of. That tension between the medical perspective that views periods of 10 or 15 years as a kidney transplantee as an achievement and the simple wish entertained by me and other transplantees to live a full, normal life after the transplant has not been resolved to this day. There are transplantees who are lasting 20 or 30 years after the transplant. Unfortunately, I do not share their good luck and my life goes from one transplant to another.

So, what now? I was 26 and my life course looked like a dead end. Again, I was facing the choice between dialysis and transplant. Another transplant. I needed another kidney. My health problems burst into the life course I had planned for myself and blew up the mask of normalcy I had worked so hard to preserve. At 26, thoughts come up that had not been there at the age of 13: what was the degree of my responsibility? Was it moral to receive more than one transplant? What would my life look like from there on, and especially the practical question: where was I going to get my lifesaving kidney?

My mother answered the question instantly and absolutely. She came forth resolutely and offered herself as a donor with no prior discussion, or at least not any to which I was party. "I felt it was my turn after Dad had donated you a kidney," she told me later. She stepped forward and with no hesitation quickly went through the compatibility tests so that I would not need even a single dialysis session before the transplant. I don't remember any hesitation or second thoughts on her part. It is hard to stop a mother who wants to save her son's life and put it back on track. Two and a half months after the conversation with the doctor, in November 1999, I went through my second transplant.

The months after the transplant were not easy. I contracted viruses and my kidney function began deteriorating quickly. Within six months, it stabilized at reasonable indexes and allowed me four and a half more years of life as a kidney transplantee. The psychological impact of the second transplant radically changed my attitude toward myself as an organ transplantee. I realized that my identity as a kidney transplantee was not an intimate detail I could hide and manage on the edges of my life. The concept of the heroism of the disabled person who "doesn't show it" became meaningless to me. It was both sobering and empowering, because from that point on I began asking myself what it meant to be a kidney transplantee.

Unlike other medical conditions, being a kidney transplantee means that the solution to your health status does not come only from the medical and pharmacological sciences, but that it is primarily dependent on your surrounding social world. In that case, what does it mean to be a trained sociologist and a kidney transplantee? For me, it was clear. It meant that I must apply the capabilities and skills I had learned, to study the world of organ transplantation from a sociological perspective. That is how my plan for the coming years became clear to me. Surely, the option of going to study in the United States was off the table, and if I were to believe the accepted career paths, my chances of getting a position and a tenure-track were also very low. Out of that understanding, and out of determination to pursue research and academic writing, I decided to write a PhD on the sociology of organ transplantation. That was what I would do to try to answer my question of what it meant to be a kidney transplantee.

I began as usual by reading what had been written in the social sciences about organ transplantation. My interpretation of that discourse can be read in the previous chapter. Here, I will add only that it was a frustrating and upsetting experience. When I read the critical texts written about transplantation medicine, I felt deep alienation: I felt that the texts had been written by healthy people for healthy people. Texts that were written from other disciplines were not critical or reflective enough about the altruism and "gift of life" discourse, and took them at face value, which I felt was too reductive.

I went to gatherings and conferences about transplantation medicine. These were mainly conferences organized as in-service training for nursing or educational staffs. The conferences repeated themselves in form and contents: they presented the medical aspect, the legal aspect, and the religious law aspect. Actually, this form is the default perspective in Israel on bioethical issues: a physician, a jurist, and a clergyman. The physician presents the wonders of technology, and the two sidekicks provide the cover of legitimacy for the technology in question. In organ transplantations, the jurist usually talked about the legal framework and what is allowed and what is forbidden, following the dichotomy derived from the ban on organ trafficking, and the rabbi (most of the conferences were for the Jewish public) came from the circles that support the definition of brain death provided by the Chief Rabbinate, and of rabbis who support organ donation (see elaboration on this matter in Chapter 6).

These conferences may have satisfied initial curiosity about transplantation, but for me, they did not even touch the main issue that concerned me: what does it mean to be an organ transplantee? Every transplantee carries within themselves a social drama that touches at the heart of the interpersonal relationship of receiving and reward. Conversations with other transplantees did not give me satisfactory answers at that time. For them, taking their medicines on time and following the doctor's orders were answer enough. When I asked them about their feelings toward the donor, most of them said they were grateful and felt responsibility toward the donor and the donation. Today, I realize that that might be a sufficient answer, and maybe the question I asked was not fair, because once one's life has been saved thanks to another, one might be rendered speechless, and all that remains is to stick to the daily routine of taking the medicine and following the instructions.

But at the time, in 1999, I was obsessed with that question. The decision to address it as a research question for my doctoral thesis felt to me at the time like the right solution for me. The discipline of disability studies was just beginning to enter social studies from the United Kingdom and the United States, and it inspired me, along with my background in feminist theory, to present my research question as a question of "situated knowledge." At that time I lay the groundwork for the thinking presented in this book: that the most urgent question is the organ shortage, and that question sends me in a materialistic direction, and that actually I am interested in the political economy of transplantation organs.

The need for a second transplant heightened the urgency of the shortage question for me. This question is never taken off the table and preoccupies transplantees and those waiting for transplants constantly. The theoretical answers to the shortage question treated altruism as a category that exists in the world, and the practical answers were public education systems to encourage organ donation. We, the transplantees and those waiting for transplants, grateful for every lifesaving organ donation, served at best as the poster images to encourage organ donation. But for me, the question of the shortage and its partial solutions opened up a wide research field, where I hoped to find more complex answers to the relations between the organ donors and us, the transplantees.

The shortage question came into sharp relief as the central axis especially following my deteriorating health status after the second transplant. I visited the nephrological clinic more frequently and met numerous transplantees, some of them in different stages of kidney rejection, trying to fend off the end, thinking about the next transplant, and trying to find themselves solutions. For us, the educational mechanisms to encourage organ donations were an important effort, but given the long transplantation waiting lists, they seemed like an all-too-distant solution. But what could be done? What action could those on the waiting list or transplantees experiencing kidney rejection take? To get angry at the indifference of people who do not sign donor cards? Every person, bioethics teaches us, has the right to their body and to decide whether to donate organs or not. We, who are waiting for a donation, are not part of the rights discourse, but of the charity and supererogation discourse. In such a world, demanding has no legitimacy, only gratitude, recognition of favor, and moral debt.

Furthermore, as transplantees, we supposedly belong to the "world of the healthy." The donation improves our quality of life and allows us a full life. We are not disabled like the visibly disabled. Our disability is not permanent or as easily defined as an essential disability. The medical guidelines and living with a suppressed immune system are too thin a foundation upon which to build a strong collective identity, sufficient only for ad hoc organizing around a desirable lifestyle. What, then, is the sociological meaning of being a kidney transplantee?

I debated that question for a long time. I felt alienated from the altruism discourse. That was not my parents' motivation to donate. I felt deep despair over the critical social sciences writing. It made me feel like an exhibit at a horror show of medicalization and capitalism. The philosophy behind the bioethics, economics, anthropology, law, and health policy – all of the writing about transplantation medicine in these disciplines felt false to the truth I felt I shared with other transplantees. It was the truth of the shortage that interrupts your life course and condemns you to death or a life of dependence on dialysis. The challenge was how to present a sociological theory of that shortage. The following chapters present the solution I found to that challenge.

3 Living and Deceased Organ Economies

Bodies and body parts

In many senses, the medical technology of the mid-20th century created an epistemological rupture: the individual in the simplest sense – the indivisible (individum) – is no longer the basic unit of analysis. The epistemological status of body tissues, organs, and body products (cells in the case of eggs) – which, thanks to the new technologies, can be preserved and then implanted, infused, or transplanted into another body – is no longer clear (Mitchell and Waldby 2008, Hacking 2006, Rajan 2006, Heath, Rapp and Taussig 2004). The advanced medical technologies granted an autonomous sphere to components – blood, reproductive cells, tissues, and organs – which were once an inseparable part of the subject and did not have separate existence from it, and this situation required the creation of normative regulation systems. The systems that were created sought to impose on this sphere rules of ownership, rights, and allocation, and this created a new ethical field (Rose and Novas 2005).

What is the meaning of the autonomous existence of these objects? What is the nature and what is the status of a body organ in the interim situation after being extracted from one body and before being implanted into another? Medicine refers to its biological features, the law refers to its legal status (often in the context of the procurement and allocation mechanisms), whereas culture seeks to conceal the disconnection that is created between the person and their body parts. The greater the autonomy of those quasi-objects – as the preservation mechanisms become more sophisticated – the more issues concerning their medical, legal, and cultural regulation arise. The gap between the subject and their body parts is becoming so obvious that one can speak about separate spheres of existence for the individual and their body parts and to the creation of a new sphere of interactions between humans and body parts, known as "biosociality" (Rabinow 2010, Gibbons and Novas 2007). Knowledge about the body puts anthropomorphic assumptions to the test, and the genetic revolution and the mapping of the human genome illustrate that clearly (Thacker 2006). So, for example, in the case of frozen embryos, and of cells that in the laboratory become immortal cells that survive long after the death of the body that produced them (Rabinow 2011, Landecker 2000). The same is true for patenting gene sequences (Jensen and Murray

DOI: 10.4324/9781003288886-5

2005), body ownership rights (Dickenson 2007), and the personal identity and genetic cargo of donated reproductive cells. All of these reside in the autonomous sphere of movement of body organs or products. Medicine's reference unit is no longer a single organism, a single person, or a single body with a single life. Now, body parts also occupy their place in the public sphere. As such, they are new public entities whose political, cultural, social, and economic status requires clarification, and this occurs in reference to their movement in space. This space opens a new ethical field that is concerned with the significance of the organ, the tissue, or the cell that migrates from one body to another. That space is the reference unit of this book.

Many theoreticians have entered this unplowed field and tried to understand how medical technologies redefine basic concepts that were considered building blocks of the very human understanding of life itself. For example, what exactly does the genetic mapping of a specific individual represent? DNA, perceived as our intimate identity card, can be conceptualized in private, personal terms of the new individualism, which is to say that the inherited genetic conglomerate is unique and singular and the basis of the modern concept of the self (Rose 2007, Gibbon and Novas 2005). But, genetic mapping can also be perceived in national terms (Tamminen and Brown 2011). Is there a common genetic profile between different ethnic groups? Racial groups? How are the genetic databases of entire populations cataloged in biobanks? (Hartigan 2013) Can the genetic profile of homogenous populations such as that of Iceland or heterogeneous populations such as that of the United States be outlined? Does a particular population have a genetic basis? Can it serve as the basis for claiming civil rights? For instance, can a genetic test prove or disprove belonging to the Jewish people and, consequently, the entitlement to citizenship in Israel? Thus, on the one hand, the genomic revolution and the new technologies that came with it have a dimension of upending the traditional definitions of personal and collective identity on the basis of nationality, class, or other social statuses and replacing them with genetically based identities that create new categories, which often highlight the arbitrariness of national, ethnic, or racial affiliation. On the other hand, genetic identities have a strong essentialist dimension, especially when they present a relatively homogenous picture of genetic origin.

Organs on the move

In light of these developments in research and in the fields of biomedicine and biotechnology, organ transplants have a special place. As aforesaid, organ transplantation poses a new challenge to anthropomorphism and the concept of individuality. But beyond the interesting anthropology that organ transplantation offers, it entails a unique set of political economy. Whereas a great deal of literature has been devoted to the anthropological element of organ transplantation, much less attention has been given to the political economy of transplanted organs. I propose combining the two dimensions and using the anthropological singularity of organ transplantation as a basic element of its political economy.

The political economy I wish to describe, therefore, is of the organs themselves, as a separate entity that is channeled, moved, and transferred from the bodies from which they are taken and to which they are transplanted. It is an economy that should be understood out of the new geometry it creates: between bodies, at varying distances from total genetic identity to total genetic strangeness, between different scales of distance – physically and socially, between intimacy and strangeness. Organ transplantation brings together body parts and persons based on tissue typing and genetic proximity and creates a new sense for sameness and otherness.

Organs for transplantation are in constant motion from one body to another. The portable fridge with "Human Organ for Transplant" printed on it is perhaps one of organ transplantations' common images. In fact, this ice box contains three bags: one for the organ immersed in preservation solution. This bag is put in a second bag with saline solution and the two bags are put in a third bag with saline. The optimal temperature for preserving the organ in its travel is between 4°C and 8°C (Michel, LaMurgalia, Madariaga and Anderson 2015). Organs for transplantations are rushed from one medical center to another, on some occasions by airplanes that take them between countries and overseas. The time during which the organ is not oxygenated by blood flow needs to be as short as possible: This is cold ischemic time and it can be no longer than 4 hours for hearts and lungs, 12–16 hours for livers, and up to 24 hours for kidneys. This is the period of time in which the organ is separated from any body, free in some sense, living on borrowed time in an ice box. This period of time is the countdown for finding – in the case of organs taken from the deceased – its recipient. This includes profiling the organ in terms of tissue typing, blood type, and antigen makeup and then finding a match from candidates on the waiting list (Maciel, Hwang and Greer 2017).

The separated life of the organ, in deceased donations, starts before its harvest and saline preservation. When consent to donation is obtained, some measures need to be taken in order to sustain the organ's vitality. The body heat is preserved by the artificial circulation of blood in the donor's body. Blood pressure is kept as well as other functions that help preserve the body. This, as argued in Chapter 1, leads to the paradoxical status of the living body of the dead donor. In this initial stage, the organ is still dependent on its original body environment. But from the moment it is disconnected from the donor's body and to the moment it is connected to the recipient's blood vessels, it is an object of its own.

During this short and quick period of time, where the organ is an object of its own, it has different statuses that determine its ontology. In the case of deceased donation, it is the healthy organ of a dead person that with its disconnect from the donor's body, the donor completes her demise. In the case of living organ donation, it is the sacrificed healthy organ of a healthy person that by her sacrifices loses something of her health.

The organ's clinical status is determined by its functional indices and its vitality. A damaged organ is disqualified for a transplant. These indices can foretell the organ's future functions in the recipient body. The organ genetic profile is an additional status beyond the clinical function. The blood type, antigen, and tissues make up point to who can be a suitable recipient of the organ.

Once a recipient is found and called for transplantation, the organ receives its biosocial status: it is from now on a designated organ; no longer body-free, but an organ with body address, body destination, and b-mail. For organs taken from living people, this body-mail is pre-set. It is the result of a long donation process of qualification tests. For organs taken from deceased persons, the body-mail is set by the chance of death.

The fifth status in the biosocial life of organs for transplantations is its ethical status. This status is dependent on the transplant context. The organ for transplant can be a token of altruism, benevolence, love, and sacrifice. In different circumstances, it can be a commodity, an organ with a fixed price, and an object that was taken by coercion and exploitation. As we shall see throughout the book, the ethical status is diversified and interdependent on the political economy that channels the organ from one body to another.

After being transplanted, the organ does not lose its former status. It has a distinct genetic makeup, different from. that of the recipient body, its clinical status is monitored routinely in hospital checkups, and it is functioning thanks to the downplaying of the host's immune system. Kidneys are transplanted in the abdominal cavity and are connected to the urine bladder and the blood system differently than they are usually. It is customary not to touch the native kidneys if there is no need. The native kidneys, due to their nonfunction, are then shrunk.

The transplanted organ still holds its biosocial and ethical statuses. We will discuss in detail these statuses and their development throughout the book. At this stage, it is sufficient to argue that these statuses are the result of the social institutions that actually provided the organ. It is here where social dispositions such as gender, family role, class, and even race play a role in the ethics of organ supply. Indeed, although organ buyers are exempted from criminal liability, they are not free from ethical responsibility. Likewise, a person who received an organ from a next of kin or a friend is caught up in the convoluted relations of family ties or friendship. Organ recipients' ethics is often reduced to the duty of keeping the organ healthy for as many years as it is possible. As we shall see later on, this ethics is only one layer in the relations between the donor and the recipient.

Transplant medicine manufactures new social configurations and cosmologies by the very travel routes of the organs from body to body. But these anthropological insights cannot be divorced from the political economy that draws these travel routes of organ parts. As argued in Chapter 1, it is the shortage of organs which is the primer of this political economy.

What is organ economy?

The perspectives of political economy or economic sociology – precisely because of their emphasis on interactions between social institutions – offer a different analytical horizon from that proposed by the ethical, legal, or the "new materialism" approach of anthropology. The analytical advantage of the approach proposed here is twofold: first of all, political economy and economic sociology are concerned with understanding the movement of goods, commodities, or any other object between social institutions. Organs' movement occurs by the mediation of social institutions. It is the state, the market, the family, or any combination of the three that make the social foundations of organ supply. Second, the motion of body organs does not occur in a vacuum but is shaped by specific social, cultural, legal, and political circumstances. Thus, it is important whether the starting point of organ transfer is in the private sphere or in the public. Political economy enables us to make a more accurate analysis of the interaction between the organ economy and social institutions. It enables us to discuss the organ economy from its material perspective – namely, from the perspective of shortage, supply, demand, and so on – without abandoning its institutional aspect, which gives the movement of organs a political, social, and cultural meaning.

Therefore, the concept of an "organ economy" is not part of the discipline of economics; it is not an expansion of the principles of classical or neoclassical economics into another domain, nor is it an exercise in game theory, cost–benefit calculations, or the pricing of shortage. An organ economy perspective views the supply system of transplantation organs as a consequence of the source of the organ (from a living or dead person); the separation between the public sphere and the private sphere; the hybrid structures on the boundary between the private and the public; and the activity of official and unofficial networks for the procurement and allocation of organs. Therefore, this is an attempt to trace the deep social structures that cause the fluctuations in the supply of organs for transplantation. Thus, for instance, one of the main questions for discussion here is the relationship between the organ economy and the weakening of the state and the rise of the ethos of individualism in neoliberal economies. In other words, the organ economy employs a classical system of categories of analysis from the field of political economy to delineate the space created by the transfer of organs from body to body and ultimately enable us to reconsider the questions of legitimacy, ethics, and morality.

In the following sections, I will draw the contours of organ political economy in a triple move. I will first discuss the dual source of organ economy (living and deceased donations), then I will delve into the triple structure of state, markets, and families as the social foundations of organ economy and conclude by drawing the four dimensions of this economy that are created by the crisscrossing of the public–private axis and the altruism–utilitarian axis. This could be read as somewhat rigid framing. However, this proposed structure enables the contextualization of moral judgments and a better understanding of where do organs come from. A more nuanced analysis, both at the global level and in specific local contexts, will be introduced in Chapter 4.

The dual source of transplantation organs

Living organ economy and deceased organ economy operate on different tracks, and they have different systems of procurement and allocation and organ provider–recipient relations. They move in different spheres of activity, which, in turn, provide them with separate ethical and moral environments.

The distinction between an organ coming from a living person (95% of all living organ donations are of a kidney) and an organ coming from a cadaver (a growing number of transplantable organs) also has medical, clinical, and ethical implications. Furthermore, it has implications for the fabric of relationships between the donor and the recipient and, again, for the way the organs are procured and allocated and the way the donation is justified.

Preparing a living organ donor includes meticulous physical and psychological checkups before qualifying someone as an organ donor (Sanner 2005). This set of check points can last for months and may slow down the process and even cool down the first enthusiasm that draws people to decide to donate their organs. It results in a more balanced view of the process and with their initial consent being comprehensively understood and informed (Henderson and Gross 2017). Conversely, check points for deceased donations run fast once death is confirmed. It includes obtaining consent, qualifying the transplantability of the deceased organs, and matching a suitable recipient from the waiting list. All of this should not take more than a few hours so that the deceased's organs will not lose their vitality. The different process of organ retrieval denotes the distinct ethical and clinical concerns of each supply source. This difference continues even after the transplant, with studies indicating long survival rates for organs taken from living donors (Nemati, Einollahi, Pezeshki et al. 2014).

As we saw in Chapter 1, the ethical justification for organ donation from the living relies on the argument of the tremendous benefit it provides – saving or improving the recipient's life – compared to the small risk of the surgery. Furthermore, it is argued that the quality of life of organ donors is even higher than average because donors aware of the risk and at peace with their decision lead healthier lifestyles than the rest of the population (Foley and Ibrahim 2010). But that finding, as encouraging as it may be, does not resolve the ethical dilemma of organ transplantations from the living: is it right to risk a healthy person in favor of another person? As argued in Chapter 1, framing the donation as "sacrifice" and as "altruistic" behavior allegedly frees the medical team from sticking to its oath. The long process of consent in living donation buttress the legitimacy to divert from the Hippocrates oath and harvest a kidney from a healthy person. Altruism here serves as a gateway from the professional ethical dilemma of doctors.

As for donation from the deceased, as discussed before, the dead donor rule was meant to resolve the challenge of the living body of the dead donor. But the definition of death, particularly brain death, turned out to be problematic, especially with the development of diagnostic technologies that discovered that brain death is more of a process than a concrete point in time and cannot be located in a single absolute point in the brain, but rather its definition requires a normative decision as to which brain function determines the end of life. But even if we accept the definition of brain death, the number of cases of brain death out of all deaths is small. Whereas the demand for organs for transplantation is growing, the number of cases of brain death is diminishing. The main causes of brain death are traffic accidents and different kinds of strokes (in fact, any direct damage to the brain). The World Health Organization reported that in 2016 stroke was one of the two leading causes of death in the world. Along with terminal heart disease, stroke has been the second cause of death in the world for the last 25 years and is measured in millions every year.[1] It was also reported that fatal traffic accidents in 2016 killed a million and a half people throughout the world. Indeed, the number of deaths from stroke and traffic accidents exceeds the demand for organs for transplantation: in the United States alone, 140,000 people die of stroke, whereas the number of people waiting for a transplant is 100,000. However, most of the deaths from stroke occur in the elderly population.[2] Furthermore, stroke is associated with vascular diseases and is common among population groups whose health is poorer than the general population. Therefore, people who die of strokes are less suitable for organ donation. On the other hand, those who are most suitable for organ donation are healthy young people who died brain death, usually in fatal traffic accidents. Luckily, improved protective measures (helmets, airbags, and more) reduce fatal head injuries, thereby reducing the number of cases of brain death among young people (Bendorf, Kerridge, Kelly et al. 2012).

A study in the United Kingdom of all cases of death recorded in ICUs in 2003–2005 found that out of 46,801 deaths, only 2,740 were identified as candidates for organ donation. Of those, only 1,244 actually donated, only 2.6% of the deaths, because not all families agreed to donate (Barber, Falvey, Hamilton et al. 2006). A more recent and comprehensive study examined the deceased donation rate in relation to brain death cases in 27 countries. It found that mortality connected with brain death decreased over years in all countries, but the utilization of brain deaths as source for organ donations vary internationally with Spain, the United States and France lead (Weiss, Elmer, Mahillo et al. 2018). These studies bring us back to the domain of the sociology of organ donation and what deter people from donation. Barriers to consent are numerous and range from trust in the medical system to opposing brain death (Moschella 2018). Studies indicate a clear sociology of reluctance to organ donations with minorities, socioeconomic disposition, and groups if color exhibits mistrust and refusal (Mohan, Muttel, Patzer et al. 2014, Patzer and McClellan 2012, Russell, Robinson, Thompson et al. 2012, Siminoff, Burnat and Ibrahim 2006, Callender and Miles 2001). Prior knowledge about organ donation increases willingness to donate (Morgan 2004), but it is associated with access to knowledge, literacy, and socioeconomic status. This matter is salient among minority groups. The access of these groups to the resources of the dominant culture is limited, and their suspicious attitude toward the establishment, including healthcare professionals, factors their reluctance to take part as organ donors. As a result, the rate of organ donations among these groups is low compared to the general population (Malek, Keys, Kumar et al. 2011). Melanson et al. (2017) point to an increase in the incidence of Hispanic and African-American patients in accessing transplantation after amending the allocation system in 2014.[3]

The state, family, and the market – the bases of organ supply

Political economy discusses the division of labor between the state and the market as economic players (Dobb 2012) [1932]. During the last decade of the last century, feminist critiques argued for expanding this dichotomy to include the family as a major player in the political economy of capitalism (O'connor, Orloff and Shaver 1999, Orloff 1993). This triangle – the state, the market, and the family – forms also the social foundation of the political economy of organs. These triple basis channel organs to transplantations through distinct routes with distinct ethical and moral envelopes. In some instances, these routes intersect each other with one basis places a checking point to a route of a different kind; sometimes, they overlap and, in some instances, they run in parallel.

The first basis is the state. It is responsible for the deceased organ economy and it operates on the public sphere with ethics that is based on autonomy, consent, fairness, and equity as well as ethical adaptation to meet the exacerbating organ shortage. The second basis is the household or the family which operates exclusively in the living organ economy and demonstrates an ethics of family relations, and the third is the illegal market of organ trafficking which introduces a violent and blunt version of businesslike ethics.

In what follow, I will define the feature of each basis of organ supply. Interestingly, the roots of this political economy, and specifically even in the terms of the political economy of organs for transplantations, can be found in Hegel. Historically, the array of moral norms of each one of the three bases was institutionalized along with the development of Capitalist political economy. The historical project of building a moral economy that would buttress the division of labor between states and markets in capitalism can be found, most explicitly, in Hegel's "Philosophy of Right" (1825). In this piece, Hegel sought to demonstrate how the ethical idea of law is fully realized in the political structure of the modern state, and to that end, he distinguishes between the normative regimes of the family, the market, and the state. He claims that the normative regime of the family is in contrast with the normative regime of the market because family relations are based on love and commitment, whereas relations in the market and civil society are utilitarian and based on interest. He claims that the market is the antithesis of the family, and dialectically the state is a synthesis of both, because it offers commitment to all (Hegel 2015). Shlomo Avineri articulated this triad in terms closer to the subject of this book: he called the normative regime Hegel attributes to the family "particular altruism," the normative regime Hegel attributes to the market "universal egoism," and the normative regime Hegel attributes to the state "universal altruism" (Avineri 1974).

Hegel's formulation does not refer, of course, to the ethics of supplying organs for transplantation, and the term "altruism" was coined decades after his death, but his theory can still be applied to the world of organ transplants. The organ economy is based on the market–family–state triad, and it too is characterized – in Avineri's terms – by the tension between altruism and utilitarianism, considerations of welfare and social rights, and the logic of the market and commerce. Hegel discusses the realization of an "ethical life," in his words, in the framework of social associations, and the state as the embodiment of the ideal of social life. For our purpose here, the importance of these things is not only the drawing of the three-way model of the political economy of organ transplants but also the delineation of the normative envelope that legitimizes three different kinds of social relations. As we shall see later, the Hegelian model largely shapes the normative expectations for each one of the tracks of the movement of organs and gives rise to the creation of hybrid structures such as family–state, market–state, and market–family. Hegel allows us to trace back the ideological roots of these moral regimes and understand how they gave rise to a series of paradoxes, as we shall see. At this stage, I wish to use the basic Hegelian model to describe in greater detail the different characteristics of each one of the three corners of the organ economy triangle. I will do it using three criteria that feature each basis: the source of the organ, the social relations, and the normative regime. These criteria will serve me later to draw the travel routes of transplantation organs according to the party who provided them and indicate the differences between these routes and the points of encounter between them.

The state

As aforesaid, the state has a monopoly on the deceased organ economy. This monopoly does not derive from the state ability to operate an intricate biopolitical bureaucracy. Extracting an organ from a cadaver and implanting it in the body of a patient require a brachiated logistical system and high organizational capacity. As described above, the time period between extracting and organ from a deceased donor and transplanting it in a recipient, an unknown recipient at the time of organ retrieval, is very short. The process must start already in ICU's with the determination of brain death, approaching the family and obtaining consent a complex and very sensitive process. Once the family's consent is obtained, a series of tests must be run for diagnosis and compatibility, to identify the most compatible patient for the transplant, the one whose body has the lowest chances of rejecting the organ.

The travel of the organs, therefore, depends on the proper functioning of the procurement mechanisms, but it is no less connected to the allocation mechanisms. Managing the transplant waiting list is a sophisticated organizational project (Zamperetti, Bellomo, Piccinni et al. 2011). The waiting list is composed on the basis of medical criteria such as the severity of the disease and its progress, and the resistance of the immune system, but also criteria on the boundary between medicine and ethics – such as prioritizing the young. But the allocation of organs for transplantation is decided primarily by the compatibility of blood type and the biological features of the donor – whose death is, of course, random and unexpected. Therefore, the deceased organ economy contains inbuilt uncertainty. The patients know what their approximate place is in the queue, but after consent to donate, the allocation mechanisms re-sort and reorder the queue. The criteria cited above are still valid, but they are categorized based on the physical characteristics of the organ: the person from which it is taken, their age, their blood type, the tissue categorization, and so on. Only a large organizational body such as a state can orchestrate the work of extraction, collection, matching, identification, and transfer of the organ within a timeframe of hours (Machado 1998).

The allocation system is supposed to be blind and neutral, but, in fact, is not. Studies in the United States, for instance, found a clear bias against African-Americans: that group was found compatible mainly for donations from African-Americans, but since the rate of donations among African-Americans is low, that group ends up deprived in terms of organ allocation. That raises suspicion and mistrust among that group toward the medical system, in general, and the transplantation system, in particular. Thus arises a closed circuit: a scarcity of organ donations from African-Americans leads to "discrimination" of patients from that group, the discrimination leads to an increase in suspicion of racial bias, and subsequently further reduces that population's willingness to donate organs. Therefore, uncertainty has a twofold impact on the deceased organ economy: it requires the existence of an organizational system able to operate effectively within a short time, and it might undermine the trust in the organ allocation mechanism.

The fact that the state has the monopoly on the transfer of organs from deceased donors and is the one who makes the rules for their procurement and allocation, which is to say the exchange rules makes it possible to provide anonymity to the parties involved. At its will, the state can share the information about the identity of the donor and the recipient with the parties involved or with the entire public, and at its will, it can keep the information confidential. Furthermore, anonymity is a condition of the procurement mechanism: the law forbids dedicating the organ donation to a particular person or a particular group. Such stipulation is a privilege of the state: only it can decide on the priorities for organ donation and the scoring system that determine one's place on the waiting list. It can be described with the help of a triad structure, in which the state connects between the giver and the recipient. This position gives the state the precedence in determining the donor of the interaction, and its power is further boosted by the anonymity of the two other parties. Thus, the deceased organ economy can be designed as an economy of social goods in which the donation is given without material stipulation. The structure of a triad characterizes also organ market economy, which also maintains the parties' anonymity and the middleman mediates the exchange.

Seemingly, transplantation medicine, in general, and the procurement of organs from the deceased, in particular, are a clear example of the biopolitics of death. The sovereignty of the state, with its administrative and organizational arms, is expressed not only by its power over its living citizens but also, mainly, according to thinker Giorgo Agamben, by its control mechanisms over the dead. In his book "Homo Sacer" (1998), Agamben presents transplantation medicine as a clear example of that control, and the brain-dead person is presented as a clear example of his concept of "exposed life" (Agamben 1998:164–165). However, contrary to Agamben's theory, which attributes to the state the supreme power both in the definition of brain death and in harvesting organs for transplantation from brain dead – the deceased organ economy actually attests to the state's weakness, and as we shall see, to impose categorically its new definition of death. Even after legalizing international brain death laws and issuing medical protocols for determining such a death, the opposition to this definition is widespread as not less fierce as it was when brain death was proclaimed at the end of the 1960s. An exception, however, is China, which, by its brutal conduct sentences, its citizens and residents to death, especially practitioners of Falun Gong, does illustrate Agamben's argument. China maintains a state-sponsored organ market and thereby creates a large reserve of organs for transplantation as state property (Matas and Kilgour 2007). But, liberal democracies find it mostly difficult to campaign for brain death as just another death and actually fail to effectively maintain the biopolitical mechanism that Agamben was afraid of.

Contrary to Agamben's model, the state does not have a free hand in organ harvesting. The state limits its powers with the consent regimes it enforces on itself, which actually gives a lot of power to the families. As we have seen above, despite the evidence of the rise in organ donations in countries that follow the presumption of consent model, most countries adhere to the informed consent model. Furthermore, most of them have a normative supervision system that seeks to ensure that organ donation is done solely out of nonmaterial motives. In the deceased organ economy, altruism is expressed mainly by adhering to the non-stipulation of the donation and its anonymity. Withdrawal from these conditions, such as in the case of increasing the social worth component of organ allocation, like a certain age group or ethnic affiliation, impedes the degree of altruism because it creates a distinction between groups and their motivations for donation can be colored by considerations of social preference. In the coming chapters, I will refer extensively to such cases and their causes.

In conclusion, the state's role in the deceased organ economy has three characteristics: (a) the state has a monopoly over the supply of deceased organs; (b) states base their organ allocation policies on different interpretations of the concept of altruism and giving, expressed by different models of consent to donate; (c) the state, as the intermediate between the donor and the recipient, guarantees to its best ability the anonymity of both. The donor cannot stipulate their donation to a certain social group or certain person, and the recipient does not know the identity of the donor. However, the state has the privilege to propose alternative standards for organ allocation and create a certain policy of stipulation of donation.

The market

Black markets of organ trafficking are an extreme case of organ economy privatization processes. The emergence of organ markets is primarily the outcome of the scarcity problem coupled with hegemony of market logics of late capitalisms and the horizons that globalization processes open for the transnational transfer of commodities, any commodities including human organs, below the inspecting eyes of the state or even international organizations. Indeed, scarcity is the engine of any market, and as long as the state of scarcity is chronic and even exacerbating, the economic stakes of trade rare goods increases. Furthermore, with prolonging scarcity, the power equation renders those who are in need, more vulnerable. In the case of end-stage patients, transplant is their only hope for restoring their health on the one side, and people whose desperation is so profound that they offer to sell one of their kidneys, organ markets are the epitome of exploitation, offense, and wrongdoing. In a series of conversations with organ vendors in Pakistan, Aamir Jafarey gives voice to their fears, trauma, and regret. None of his interviewees recommend on selling a kidney, none of them gain riches, and all of them still struggle with poverty and financial difficulties (Rippon 2014, Jafarey 2009, Cohen 2001, Schepher Hughes 2001). Exploring practices of organ trafficking in Colombia, Mendoza (2010) provides interesting data from 151 organ vendors in Bogota and Medellin. His research introduces the vendors' sociodemographic profile: they are mostly men (80.8%), between 20 and 40 years of age (74.2%), occupy low (55%) and lowest (31%) income stratum, are either single with dependents (42.4%) or married with dependents (45%), and half of them (51%) attended secondary school. This profile tells a story of disempowered persons with responsibility to their dependents that are pushed to the point of despair. Mendoza also discovers what was their point of entry to the organ market: 32% of them initiated the selling of an organ, 40% received recommendation on selling an organ from family members and friends, and 28% were approached by a third party, i.e., doctors, agencies, or syndicates. Sixty percent of the vendors received 1,000–2,000 US$ and they reported to the researchers that their aim was immediate cash.[4]

It is self-evident that organ markets are not markets in the classical economic sense. According to the accepted definition, normative markets are based on free will, transparency, and accountability. These features certainly do not exist in actual organ markets. Indeed, proponents of regulated organ markets invest efforts to tailor an appearance of a free, accountable, transparent, and even moral markets. But, in contrast to these theoretical discussions, the actual organ market – illegal and operated underground – are a place of fraudulent, cynical, and offensive. In fact, the organ markets are a reverse mirror image of the market in its classical definition. They have neither free will in the full sense of the word nor transparency, and they certainly have no accountable guarantees. Yet, organ markets are an important locus in the political economy of organ supply, mostly of kidneys.

Most of the organ markets are kidney markets. Extracting and transplanting a kidney are relatively simple procedures that do not require particularly sophisticated surgical theaters and from which recovery is relatively quick, and therefore, they are easier to perform underground. Organ markets operate in an economic climate of neoliberalism and globalization: the neoliberalism provides a moral cover for the utilitarian discourse, and the globalization provides refuge from state sovereignty and the moral economy of altruism it imposes. Melinda Cooper suggests looking at the development of medical technologies as wholly derived from neoliberal ideology. The very pricing and commercializing of genetic information at the cellular level is an indication of neoliberal logic as the key to understanding the new life technology industry (Cooper 2011). Not only the commercialization of body parts, tissue, and cells are part of "the new economy" at the turn of the century, but also the liberal concept of autonomy that underlies bioethics today goes hand in hand with these processes of marketization. From this perspective, it seems as the development of organ markets is almost self-evident. The question then is not about the logic of organ markets but about the logic that forbids them.

Interestingly, when going underground, scarcity or shortage is replaced by abundance of poverty and despair. In the underground organ markets, the waiting lists are not just of patients waiting for transplants, but of people from disempowered groups waiting to sell their organs.[5] The stark contrast between the existing shortage and what proponents of organ markets see as a potential of closing this shortage with commercial organs leads to the argument that not only organ markets are more effective but also more moral (Cherry 2015). Drawing their arguments upon the core values of liberalism, proponents of organ markets defend the autonomy of an individual to sell her body parts and call for a regulated market that will protect the seller's health.[6]

Most of the countries in the world forbid organ trafficking with different levels of enforcement. As altruism became the yardstick of organ donation worldwide, the trafficking of organs was outlawed and is perceived as one of the most egregious wrongs, and the war against it is waged by international bodies, physicians' associations, and health agencies. The combat against organ trafficking and organ markets is old as the technique of transplantation medicine. The idea of supplying organs through a market system remained always at the theoretical level and never materialized (except in Iran). With the intensification of globalization processes during the 1990s, the global market of organ trafficking expanded and developed, exploiting the poverty of the global south for the benefit of desperate patients, mainly from the global north. An important landmark in the war is the 2008 Declaration of Istanbul on Organ Trafficking and Transplant Tourism. The declaration is a joint international project by the Transplantation Society and the International Society of Nephrology (ISN). It brought together representatives of physicians and official transplant organizations from more than 100 countries to publicly denounce organ trafficking and contains clear recommendations for legislation outlawing it. Since the declaration was published, clear laws against organ trafficking were passed and loopholes in existing laws were closed. The war on organ trafficking takes place mainly on the legal level. As part of this war, physicians suspected of involvement in organ trafficking are indicted and international arrest orders are issued against suspects in brokering such trafficking, in an attempt to overcome the evasiveness and secrecy of those involved.

It is hard to estimate the extent of organ trafficking in the illegal markets, but very conservative estimates are of thousands of organs per year, whereas other estimates put it at tens of thousands of cases, mainly in the Chinese organ market – even if the phenomenon has lessened since the Istanbul Declaration.[7] The WHO report on global organ trafficking is from 2007, and certainly, the picture has changes given the international combat on organ markets and the Istanbul declaration (López-Fraga, Domínguez-Gil, Capron, et al. 2014, Epstein and Danovitch

2013). A distinction between the trafficking of living organs (kidneys) and the trafficking of deceased persons' organs must be drawn in order to identify state run markets. These markets operate under the auspice of the state. As mentioned, the deceased organ economy needs a formal auspice that is able to provide the necessary logistical array. Of course, most organ markets lack access to that array, but there are exceptions.

In cases of cooperation between the state and the market, the organ market will operate in the form of medical tourism, in which healthcare services are offered to economically able patients. In China, as described above, prisoners have been executed and some of their organs have been harvested for transplantation, usually in the bodies of patients outside of China (Caplan, Danovitch, Shapiro et al. 2011, Matas and Kilgour 2007). That is an example of a market operated directly by the state, whose profits flow into its treasury and were condemned time and again by the international medical community (Trey, Sharif, Schwarz et al. 2016).

The picture is a little different when it comes to trafficking in living organs. In this case, the market operates under the protection that the political economy has given to donations between living relatives. Thanks to the pharmacological progress concerning managing the immune system reaction, genetic incompatibility can be overcome and organs can be transplanted between strangers with a high level of success. This has greatly expanded the potential circles of donors for each patient, and today, a person can receive a donation even without full genetic compatibility – from a partner, a friend, an acquaintance, or a stranger. This opens a wider range of possibilities for organ trafficking. Mary Andre Jacob showed how organ markets operate under the guise of a friendly or familial relationship with the patient and traced the way organ sellers pose as distant relatives in order to "donate" an organ (Jacob 2012).

Despite the essential difference between the state's altruistic model and the market economy concerning the organ economy, there are several lines of similarity between them. Both of these organ economies are structured as triads: the organ supplier, the organ recipient, and a mediating party (transplant coordinator or alternatively organ broker). The mediating party has a critical importance in shaping the interaction between the parties and actually controls the two other parties. Likewise, in both organ economies, the anonymity of the sides is maintained. In the official organ economy, anonymity is required by the policy of altruism. In the market economy, anonymity is important to give the exchange an appearance of a businesslike transaction, in which personal profit serves as the only and exclusive interest of the participants in the interaction, just like any supposedly objective exchange between seller and buyer in any market. Like in any exchange transaction, immediately after the transaction, each side retreats back into their private, sheltered world, without knowledge about the other side. The terms "free will," "transaction," and "personal profit" characterize the neoliberal economy and also serve in the organ market in such a way that covers the exploitation, the coercion, the deceit, and the harm that are common in that market.

The family

The family as a source of organ supply became evident with the first successful kidney transplant in 1954 performed by Joseph Murrey. It was a transplant of a kidney between twins and the genetic identity proved how genetic proximity is crucial for the reception of the graft in the host body. This achievement marked genetically related family members as the ultimate pool of kidney donors for the evolving and then futuristic medical technology. Genetic proximity, however, entailed a distinct sociological and ethical conception of donation. The donation cannot be anonymous but rather directed to a specific patient, a family member who meets genetic criteria for best matching. This direct donation is a living donation. Family members donate kidneys (seldom liver lobes) to their relatives with maximizing chances of transplant timing and outcome. Direct donations in families often turn this channel of organ supply to somewhat akin to a household economy.

The household economy of organ supply is distinctive from the state channels of supply or the market underground routes of organ selling in three ways. First, the household organ economy is set on the suture between the private and the public. On the one hand, the intrafamilial dynamic that leads to donation is not under the state's control and is locked within the boundaries of the private sphere. On the other hand, organ transplantation between relatives requires the approval of the state and cannot be performed until it is validated as legitimate. Furthermore, while the state is allowed to disqualify the donation, it is not a partner in finding the actual donor in the family. This is a mission imposed on the patient and her family. The whole initiative for finding a donor is entangled in family ties and relations that constitute the "household organ economy."[8]

A second distinction concerns the moral envelope of altruism that is attached to donations between family members. This moral stamp from common beliefs on sacrifice, usually of parents to their children or brother/sisterhood between siblings or gratitude of children to their parents. These motives do exist, but they do not exhaust the wide range of relations between family members that may lead to donation. There are mounting testimonies of donations that result from intrafamilial dynamics involving power relations, coercion, and exploitation, especially of women (Gill and Lowes 2008, Crombie and Franklin 2006, Biller-Andorno 2002). In such cases, even if the donation is made out of genuine concern for the patient, it is far from being purely altruistic. In fact, it is hard to speak about altruism within nuclear family where relations are intense and continuous. The household economy is concealed behind the curtain of privacy and intimacy. An empirical evidence of the power relations that dominate the household economy of organ donation is the persistent gender gap where it is more women that donate than men to their family members (Crowley-Matoka 2016).

Household organ economy is distinct from the market and the state supply channels in its donors' type diversity and their respective relations to the patient. While the deceased donation that the state provides is of a subject who wished to donate her post-mortem body to an anonymous stranger and the kidney vendor is motivated by financial incentives, the familial donation can be motivated by very different stories. Spousal donation is different than sibling donation which is different from parental donation. All exhibit different interpersonal relations between the donor and the recipient that date long back since the need for a donation has emerged. In that sense, family organ supply resembles household economy in its emotional economy and power structure that determines the division of labor, care, and duties.

As aforesaid, both the deceased organ economy and the living organ economy mediated by the black market are characterized by anonymity and indirect donation. In contrast, the intrafamilial organ economy is characterized by a lack of anonymity and directed donation. In fact, the state and the family are at odds when it comes to the assumptions of their social relationships: the deceased organ economy mediated by the state is based on the relationship between the individual and society, and the donor is usually a stranger and anonymous. Inside a family, in contrast, strangeness and anonymity are undesirable and even fundamentally rejected. To the contrary, the main interest of the evaluation committees is the examination of the relationship between the donor and the recipient. At question is a direct donation designated for a specific patient – from mother to son, from daughter to father, and from nephew to aunt. Donation within the family by definition cannot be considered completely altruistic because altruism requires giving to a stranger, unconditionally. Unlike the deceased organ economy, in which the organs are social goods provided by the state, in an economy where the source of the organ is a relative, the organs are personal, direct, and subjective gifts.

The anonymous living donor, a person wishing to donate an organ from their body to a needy stranger without identifying themselves, may express the highest level of altruism, but such donation is not consistent with the assumption of donation from a living person. The prevailing assumption is that there are close relations between the giver and the recipient and that the organ donation is the consequence of close acquaintance, intimacy, and, sometimes, cohabitation. As we shall see in the final chapter, the anonymous living donor challenges the existing ethical order, in which altruism is expressed by donation from a family member or donation from the deceased.

Like the categories of the market and the state, the family as well is a dynamic category, and it is expanding with the progress of pharmacology. New drugs that more effectively suppress the immune system make it possible to constantly widen the circle of potential donors. In the past, first-degree blood relationship and genetic likeness were the best predictors of the success of a transplant because the chances the body would reject the transplanted organ were lower. In fact, at the inception of transplantation medicine, almost absolute genetic identity was needed between donor and recipient. With the progress of knowledge and technology, the demand for genetic identity was replaced by a demand of familial resemblance and added to the circle of potential donors were first-degree relatives with genetic proximity: siblings, parents, and children. Eventually, donations became possible from first-degree relatives who are not genetically related to the patient, especially partners. Thus, the boundary between relative and stranger became mostly normative, not genetic. Into the family circle in which altruistic donation is acceptable entered also partners, aunts and uncles, and nieces and nephews. Yet, more distant relatives with only an indirect relationship to the patient are suspected of ulterior motives. As the family category expands the altruistic code weakens, the concept of kinship expands so much that it is not clear to what extent the concepts of family and the altruistic stamp imprinted on it still express the primal drive to donate organs between relatives as in a three-generation nuclear family and second-degree kinship at most. Thus, the very concept of altruism expands to encompass more diverse concepts of relationship. Moreover, expanding the concept of the family also means expanding the possibilities of organ donation as a result of the use of power, exploitation, and coercion.

The flexibility in the concept of the family is not observed only in the area of organ transplantation. The split between the concept of the family and the concept of kinship, between social parenting and biological parenting, exists in almost all of the options that reproduction technologies offer today (Franklin 2013:376). In vitro fertilization, surrogacy, egg and sperm donations, and more and more fertility technologies unravel the traditional concept of family and present possibilities of kinship that are not related to genetic relationship. On the other hand, it could be argued that these technologies, with all of the diverse forms of family they allow, only reinforce the family as a dominant social institution whose realization in one form or another is impervious to almost any excuse.

The image of familyhood advanced by transplantation medicine is clearly associated with the new concept of familyhood advanced by medical technologies. In living organ economy, the family expands beyond the boundaries of its genetic sphere and includes first spouses, more distant relatives, and, finally, even friends or complete strangers. Genetic distance is transformed to social kinship under the concept of the family. Even those who are not directly included under that concept, complete strangers, who donated to strangers, become after the act a part of the receiving family. It is possible, as we shall see in Chapters 5 and 6, that even complete strangers prefer to donate as part of the concept of extended, almost tribal familyhood, to those who are like them and thereby raise another interesting aspect through which to think about the family. Ultimately, despite the long existence of the institution of family and household in the social and political order, organ transplants, like other advanced medical technologies, both undermine, expand, and change the concept of family, and also, in the same breath, reinforce and recreate that ancient institution as a central social institution in our reality.

The three-way model – state–family–market – is a correction of the classical dual model, private–public, which overlaps with the division between the state and the market or between political society and civil society. Feminist criticism of the classical model pointed to the hidden role of the family or the household in the economy. The household economy plays a central role in the political economy of welfare. The sociologist Gøsta Esping-Andersen, in his analysis of the welfare states in the postindustrial Western world, writes this:

The family is a significant player whose decisions and behavior directly impact the welfare state and the labor market, and are also influenced by them. The welfare regime should be identified more systematically with the interaction between the state, the market and the family.

Esping-Andersen indicates a model of welfare regimes that rely on the family, and more specifically, on the unpaid labor of mothers, daughters, and women, in general. He finds that this model is particularly widespread in "family-oriented" countries in southern Europe (especially in the Catholic countries). In the area of health, this assertion is even more valid because the family plays an important role in carrying the burden of care for a sick relative. The political analysis of the health economy views the expanding roles of the family as a result of the shrinking of the welfare state. The family is, therefore, a semi-official player in health policy: the state gives it responsibility and views it as an obvious and natural partner in carrying the burden of care but does not recognize the economic value of the work it performs. Therefore, the family is not a party that can be ignored in a comprehensive economic analysis. The empirical challenge is to examine the dynamic created between the family, the market, and the state, while examining how failures in one economic sphere impact the functioning of another economic sphere.

As part of regulating the relationship between the market and the state, many areas of welfare may remain without institutional patronage or with limited and weak patronage. In these cases, when the state and the market do not have the interest, ability, or permission to act, the family is forced to act as an agent of welfare. The social consequences of this development are very significant. Not only is the family not officially authorized to treat its needy member, but that work – like almost all of the work of the household and family – is not priced and its value is not calculated. In others words, the work of the family's welfare is transparent work. Furthermore, it is usually imposed on women: it is usually the mother, the daughter, or the sister who is expected to carry the burden of care (Crowley-Matoka 2016). To this is added to the burden of transparent work performed by women, which remains outside of formal cost calculations. The importance of the family according to the contemporary models of division between the private and the public is emphasized here because the family is occupying an ever-growing role in political economics, including in supplying organs for donation. As we shall see below, gender inequality also characterizes the role of the family in the organ economy.

Notes

1   http://www.who.int/en/news-room/fact-sheets/detail/the-top-10-causes-of-death.
2   https://www.cdc.gov/nchs/data/hus/hus16.pdf#023.
3   They explain the relative low representation of African American among organ recipients by a structural discrimination:

> Racial/ethnic disparities affecting blacks and Hispanics exist at each step of the
> kidney transplant process, with members of minority groups on average being less

likely to complete the necessary medical evaluation, be placed on the national waiting list, and receive a transplant. A number of characteristics of health care systems, patients, and providers are correlated to these disparities, including poverty limited numbers of dialysis facility staff members to educate patients about transplantation, physician bias, and inequitable federal policies that guide US organ allocation.

See also: Melanson, Hockenberry, Plantinga et al. (2017)

4   For a comprehensive literature review and ethical appraisal on organ trafficking, see The HOTT Project (2014). Available online: http://hottproject.com/userfiles/HOTT Project-TraffickinginHumanBeingsforthePurposeofOrganRemoval-AComprehensive LiteratureReview-OnlinePublication.pdf.
5   The lengthy waiting lists for organ transplantations are replaced by short period of waiting, especially in the case of kidneys from living sellers, which compose the bulk of organ markets (Rippon 2014).
6   A similar argumentation about autonomy is made in favor of prostitution's institutionalization.
7   https://www.who.int/bulletin/volumes/85/12/06-039370/en/.
8   In Israel, the prioritization model exhibits another twist of the public–private nexus of household organ economy: family members get extra points on the waiting list when one of them is signed on donor card. This policy renders the household economy of organ supply beneficial to all household members. See more on Chapter 6.

References

Agamben, G. (1998). *Homo Sacer: Sovereign Power and Bare Life*, Stanford: Stanford University Press.
Avineri, S. (1974). *Hegel's Theory of the Modern State*, Cambridge: Cambridge University Press.
Barber, K., Falvey, S., Hamilton, C., Collett, D., & Rudge, C. (2006). Potential for organ donation in the United Kingdom: Audit of intensive care records. *BMJ*, 332(7550), 1124–1127.
Bendorf, A., Kerridge, I. H., Kelly, P. J., Pussell, B., & Guasch, X. (2012). Explaining failure through success: A critical analysis of reduction in road and stroke deaths as an explanation for Australia's low deceased organ donation rates. *Internal Medicine Journal*, 42(8), 866–873.
Biller-Andorno, N. (2002). Gender imbalance in living organ donation. *Medicine, Health Care and Philosophy*, 5(2), 199–203.
Caplan, A. L., Danovitch, G., Shapiro, M., Lavee, J., & Epstein, M. (2011). Time for a boycott of Chinese science and medicine pertaining to organ transplantation. *The Lancet*, 378(9798), 1218.
Callender, C. O., & Miles, P. V. (2001). Obstacles to organ donation in ethnic minorities. *Pediatric Transplantation*, 5(6), 383–385.
Cherry, M. J. (2015). *Kidney for Sale by Owner: Human Organs, Transplantation, and the Market*, Washington, DC: Georgetown University Press.
Cohen, L. (2001). The other kidney: Biopolitics beyond recognition. *Body & Society*, 7(2–3), 9–29.
Cooper, M. E. (2011). *Life as surplus: Biotechnology and Capitalism in the Neoliberal Era*, Washington, DC: University of Washington Press.
Crombie, A. K., & Franklin, P. M. (2006). Family issues implicit in living donation. *Mortality*, 11(2), 196–210.

Crowley-Matoka, M. (2016). *Domesticating Organ Transplant, Familial Sacrifice and National Aspirations in Mexico*, Durham, NC: Duke University Press.

Dickenson, D. (2007) *Property in the Body: Feminist Perspectives*, Cambridge and New York: Cambridge University Press.

Dobb, M. (2012) [1937]. *Political Economy and Capitalism: Some Essays in Economic Tradition*, London and New York: Routledge.

Epstein, M., & Danovitch, G. (2013). Organ donation and organ trafficking: from dangerous anarchy to problematic equilibrium. *Paediatrics and Child Health*, 23(11), 492–496.

Foley, R. N., & Ibrahim, H. N. (2010). Long-term outcomes of kidney donors. *Current Opinion in Nephrology and Hypertension*, 19(2), 129–133.

Franklin, S. (2013). *Biological Relatives: IVF, Stem Cells and the Future of Kinship*, Durham, NC: Duke University Press.

Gibbon, S., & Novas, C. (2007). *Biosocialities, Genetics and the Social Sciences: Making Biologies and Identities*, Abington and New York: Routledge.

Gill, P., & Lowes, L. (2008). Gift exchange and organ donation: Donor and recipient experiences of live related kidney transplantation. *International Journal of Nursing Studies*, 45(11), 1607–1617.

Hacking, I. (2006). Genetics, biosocial groups and the future of identity. *Daedalus*, 135(4), 81–95.

Hartigan, J. (2013). Mexican genomics and the roots of racial thinking. *Cultural Anthropology*, 28(3), 372–395.

Heath, D., Rapp, R., & Taussig, K. S. (2004). Genetic citizenship. *A Companion to the Anthropology of Politics*, 152–167.

Hegel, G. W. F. (2015) [1825]. *The Philosophy of Right*, Indianapolis, IN: Hackett Publishing.

Henderson, M. L., & Gross, J. A. (2017). Living organ donation and informed consent in the United States: Strategies to improve the process. *The Journal of Law, Medicine & Ethics*, 45(1), 66–76.

Jacob, M. A. (2012). *Matching Organs with Donors: Legality and Kinship in Transplants*, Philadelphia, PA: University of Pennsylvania Press.

Jafarey, A. (2009). Conversations with kidney vendors in Pakistan: An ethnographic study. *Hastings Center Report*, 39(3), 29–44.

Jensen, K., & Murray, F. (2005). Intellectual property landscape for human genome. *Science*, 310(5746), 239–240.

Landecker, H. (2000). "Immortality, in vitro: A history of the HeLa Cell Line", in P. E. Brodwin (ed). *Biotechnology and Culture: Bodies, Anxieties, Ethics*, Bloomington: Indiana University Press. pp. 53–72.

López-Fraga, M., Domínguez-Gil, B., Capron, A. M. et al. (2014). A needed convention against trafficking in human organs. *The Lancet*, 383(9936), 2187–2189.

Machado, N. (1998). *Using the Bodies of the Dead: Legal, Ethical and Organisational Dimensions of Organ Transplantation*, London and New York: Routledge.

Maciel, C. B., Hwang, D. Y., & Greer, D. M. (2017). "Organ donation protocols", in *Handbook of Clinical Neurology*, Vol. 140. Elsevier. pp. 409–439.

Malek, S. K., Keys, B. J., Kumar, S. et al. (2011). Racial and ethnic disparities in kidney transplantation. *Transplant International*, 24(5), 419–424.

Matas, D., & Kilgour, D. (2007). *Bloody Harvest. Revised Report into Allegations of Organ Harvesting of Falun Gong Pratictioners in China*, 31.

Melanson, T. A., Hockenberry, J. M., Plantinga, L. et al. (2017). New kidney allocation system associated with increased rates of transplants among black and Hispanic patients. *Health Affairs*, 36(6), 1078–1085.

Mendoza, R. L (2010). Colombia's organ trade: Evidence from Bogotá and Medellín. *Journal of Public Health*, 18, 375–384.

Michel, S. G., LaMuraglia II, G. M., Madariaga, M. L. L. et al. (2015). Innovative cold storage of donor organs using the Paragonix Sherpa Pak™ devices. *Heart, Lung and Vessels*, 7(3), 246.

Mitchell, R., & Waldby, C. (2008) *Tissue Economies: Blood, Organs and Cell Lines in Late Capitalism*, Durham, NC: Duke University Press.

Mohan, S., Mutell, R., Patzer, R. E. et al. (2014). Kidney transplantation and the intensity of poverty in the contiguous United States. *Transplantation*, 98(6), 640.

Morgan, S. E. (2004). The power of talk: African Americans' communication with family members about organ donation and its impact on the willingness to donate organs. *Journal of Social and Personal Relationships*, 21(1), 112–124.

Moschella, M. (2018). "Brain death and organ donation: A crisis of public trust. *Christian Bioethics*, 24(2), 133–150.

Nemati, E., Einollahi, B., Pezeshki, M. L. et al. Does kidney transplantation with deceased or living donor affect graft survival?. *Nephro-Urology Monthly*, 6(4), e12182.

O'Connor, J. S., Orloff, A. S., & Shaver, S. (1999). *States, Markets, Families: Gender, Liberalism and Social Policy in Australia, Canada, Great Britain and the United States*, Cambridge University Press.

Orloff, A. S. (1993). Gender and the social rights of citizenship: The comparative analysis of gender relations and welfare states. *American Sociological Review*, 58(3), 303–328;

Patzer, R. E., & McClellan, W. M. (2012). Influence of race, ethnicity and socioeconomic status on kidney disease. *Nature Reviews Nephrology*, 8(9), 533.

Rabinow, P. (2011). *Making PCR: A Story of Biotechnology*, Chicago, IL: Chicago University Press.

Rabinow, P. (2010). Artificiality and Enlightenment: from Sociobiology to Biosociality. *Politix*, 2, 21–46.

Rajan, K. S. (2006). *Biocapital: The Constitution of Postgenomic Life*, Durham, NC: Duke University Press.

Rippon, S. (2014). Imposing options on people in poverty: The harm of a live donor organ market. *Journal of Medical Ethics*, 40(3), 145–150.

Rose, N., and Novas, C. (2005). Biological citizenship. In Ong, A & Collier S.J. (eds). *Global assemblages: Technology, Politics, and Ethics as Anthropological Problems*, Oxford: Blackwell Publishing, 439–463.

Rose, N. (2007) Mollecular biopolitics, somatic ethics and the spirit of biocapital. *Social Theory and Health*, 5(1), 3–29.

Russell, E., Robinson, D. H., Thompson, N. J. et al. (2012). Distrust in the healthcare system and organ donation intentions among African Americans. *Journal of Community Health*, 37(1), 40–47.

Sanner, M. A. (2005). The donation process of living kidney donors. *Nephrology Dialysis Transplantation*, 20(8), 1707–1713.

Scheper-Hughes, N. (2001). Bodies for sale–whole or in parts. *Body & Society*, 7(2–3), 1–8.

Siminoff, L. A., Burant, C. J., & Ibrahim, S. A. (2006). Racial disparities in preferences and perceptions regarding organ donation. *Journal of General Internal Medicine*, 21(9), 995–1000.

Tamminen, S., & Brown, N. (2011). Nativitas: Capitalizing genetic nationhood. *New Genetics and Society*, 30(1), 73–99.

Thacker, E. (2006). *The Global Genome: Biotechnology, Politics and Culture*, Cambridge, MA: MIT Press.

Trey, T., Sharif, A., Schwarz, A., Fiatarone Singh, M., & Lavee, J. (2016). Transplant medicine in China: Need for transparency and international scrutiny remains. *American Journal of Transplantation*, 16(11), 3115–3120.

Weiss, J., Elmer, A., Mahíllo, B., et al. (2018). Evolution of deceased organ donation activity versus efficiency over a 15-year period: an international comparison. *Transplantation*, 102(10), 1768–1778.

Zamperetti, N., Bellomo, R., Piccinni, P. et al. (2011). Reflections on transplantation waiting lists. *The Lancet*, 378(9791), 632–635.

Istanbul 2004

There are moments when everything becomes clear and lucid and reality comes into sharp, unmistakable relief. Such a moment occurred for me in July 2004. I remember the blinding sunlight that blurred the sight of the fan of cables suspending the bridge over the Bosphorus Straits, on the way from my hotel on the Asian side of Istanbul to the hidden hospital on the European side. We drove in silence. Next to me sat a hefty man, a diabetic suffering from kidney failure. The port on his arm connected his artery to his vein for his dialysis treatments. I had a tube running from below my left shoulder directly to my heart, also for dialysis. It was a Friday. The city was boisterous, hustling, and bustling, with sounds of the market and commerce mingling with the muezzin's calls to prayer. The din of the city reached our ears even when the taxi turned off the main roads and wended its way through the narrow streets of the city's outskirts. I did not know where we were going, but the situation was crystal clear: I was about to buy a kidney. The decision had been made, the preparations had begun, and there was no way back. Somebody was already lying on the operating table, waiting for their kidney to be extracted and implanted in my body, in exchange for money. It was a terrible thing to do, and here, I was doing it.

More than guilt, I was consumed with a feeling of helplessness. I was struck by the realization that there are powers stronger than ourselves that guide us to predetermined paths. Free will? Responsibility? Choice? All those words rang hollow to me, unreal in the face of the reality of my life: I was 31, married, and childless. Based on the organ waiting lists in Israel, my dialysis treatments were supposed to go on for at least five years. Dialysis may have been the moral solution, but it would have ruined my life, my wife's, and my whole family's. Would we be able to have children? Could I still work? Could I continue my academic career? My choices were stark: to stick by my values and condemn myself and my family to live under the heavy shadow of dialysis – or, conversely, to betray my values and buy a kidney for money.

I had made my choice and here was the result, materializing before my eyes. I was sitting in a taxi, on the way to a makeshift hospital in faraway Istanbul. I had bought an organ of a living person. That was the naked truth. In the face

DOI: 10.4324/9781003288886-6

of that truth, any number of words, deliberations, and thoughts are rendered moot. They crash and scatter into oblivion. I remembered the words of Nancy Scheper-Hughes: "Several key words in organ transplantation require radical deconstruction. Among them are 'scarcity,' 'need,' 'donation,' 'gift,' 'bond,' 'life,' 'death, 'supply,' and 'demand.'" What is radical deconstruction? As far as I was concerned, the situation was starkly clear. At that moment, all ideologies and all opinions about organ transplants, whether utopian or dystopian, simply collapse. Out of the ruins of morality and reason emerges the grim reality of distress.

The guy who sold me his kidney was 23. Israeli, like me. I found him following compatibility evaluation tests. Actually, his older brother was the one who was supposed to sell me a kidney. We were supposed to fly to Turkey a few weeks earlier, but at the last minute, when I was already at the entrance to the airport, I was informed he had changed his mind. Later, I learned that he too ultimately sold his kidney. They were both the sons of a grocer who had recently passed away and left behind him enormous debts to Social Security. They lived in a southern town. In that town, selling kidneys was so common in the early millennium that its residents nicknamed it "kidneytown." So, the brothers sold their kidneys to pay their late father's debt to Social Security. How ironic: I was buying an organ in order to pay off a debt to the government. I paid $100,000 for the kidney, but, of course, the full sum did not go to its owner. After the surgery, the seller told me that after a tough negotiation with the organ dealer it was agreed that he would receive $15,000. The rest of the money would be divided between those involved in the transaction, including the dealer and the surgeon.

Finally, we stopped in front of what looked like a run-down house. A nondescript house in the middle of the street, three stories of peeling plaster in the middle of one of Istanbul's outlying neighborhoods, no different from any other house on the block. Nothing disclosed what was happening inside. A black motorcycle was parked at the entrance. A narrow path led us around the house, to the back door, and from there, we were brought into the clinic, which also looked old and decrepit. I learned that this clinic was well known to Israeli kidney patients, and apparently, most of the buyers and sellers there came from Israel. The dealers, the clinic directors, the doctors, and the surgeons were Turkish and Israeli. A few years later, in 2007, I read in the newspaper that the clinic had been exposed following a robbery attempt. A gang of robbers broke into the house, police arrived, and a shootout ensued. That very day, all the doctors, the buyers, and the sellers were arrested, and the clinic's activity was stopped.

As we entered, we were led to the hospitalization room, the one devoted to the buyers. The sellers were given a separate room. As opposed to the somewhat grungy appearance of the hallway, and the joint bathrooms with their rusty faucets and shabby tiles, the hospitalization rooms looked modern and spiffy. They were illuminated with white fluorescent light that gave them an aura of faux cleanliness, which gleamed in contrast with the dim lighting of the rest of the clinic. We were required to sign a false statement to the Turkish health authorities declaring that the donation was altruistic and that there was an acquaintanceship between myself and the "donor." The rules were laid out: I would be allowed seven days of recovery. The next Friday morning, I would get on a plane to Israel, regardless of my medical condition: whether the kidney was accepted or not, whether my body was strong enough to withstand the strain of travel or not. During the recovery days, only half an hour of visits a day would be allowed, and I must be as quiet as possible so that the medical goings-on would not be discovered beyond the walls of the hidden clinic. At noon that day, I was taken up to the second floor that housed the operating rooms and underwent the transplant. It was my third transplant, this time a transplant of a traded kidney.

As mentioned, I had received the previous two kidneys from my parents. This time my search field was different. Instead of looking upward, as a child looking at his parents for answers, I had to look around me, at my own age group, at my peers. But how can you ask someone for a kidney? It is a silent request that reverberates by the very deterioration of my medical condition. In our modern neo-liberal way of life, which glorifies individualism and personal autonomy, needing charity to save your life feels like self-effacement, defeatism, and helplessness. I couldn't ask anyone. In the early millennium, before the popularization of Facebook and other social media, it was not yet possible to share my predicament safely behind a screen and keyboard. I had to actively approach people, and merely asking seemed to me like coercing the person I asked. Because how can you say no to someone who asks you to save their life?

Only after the transplant did I meet the young man who had sold me a kidney, and that is when I learned about him, his brother, and the debt to Social Security. Next to us was another pair of buyers and sellers. The buyer was an older and large man who had ridden with me in the taxi, whose kidneys had deteriorated because of diabetes. The seller was a young man. Both were Israeli. The seller received only $10,000 for his kidney. He had traveled to Turkey under the guise of a holiday, and in long phone calls reported to his relatives in Israel about his supposed travel to Turkey. At one point in one of the phone calls, he broke down and told them he had sold a kidney and was in a sort of clinic in Istanbul. At that moment, the organ dealer emerged as a violent thug and threatened him not to disclose the location of the clinic. While we were there together, the young man told me he was a gambler who got into debt and that he was selling his kidney, so he could pay his debts. But he didn't say he was going to stop gambling. His decision to sell his kidney was surely hasty and irresponsible.

Had I paid with a currency of morals for living time? Many people think that anyone would make such a deal to save their life. But that common opinion, which is socially sanctioned, actually legitimizes the exploitation, coercion, and deceit of those who are compelled to sell their organs. Some claim that these transactions demonstrate the gap between the rich, who buy organs for themselves, and the poor, who sell their organs to survive. Indeed, it is a most disgraceful trade, but as a matter of fact, it is not a question of rich versus poor, but sick versus poor. This correction has ethical significance. I saw with my own eyes the desperate attempts of many patients to raise the money needed for a transplant, whether through fundraising events or over the social networks. In fact, those efforts are more successful than you would expect. The more correct definition when it comes to organ trading is that sick people buy from poor people. Indeed, these are two groups pushed by despair into organ trading.

The long wait for an organ pushed me, as it did other patients, into the market. There I was exposed to a long list of organ sellers, longer than you can imagine. I went through compatibility tests with six or seven candidates. The only thing I knew about them was their blood type and other biological and medical data. Meanwhile, my condition continued to deteriorate. My wife volunteered to donate a kidney to me, but our blood types were not compatible. We thought about a paired exchange, in which we would find a couple, one healthy and one sick, with compatible blood types: the healthy one would donate their kidney to me, whereas my wife would donate a kidney to the sick member of the other couple. But at the time, in 2004, paired exchanges were not yet familiar and supported by transplant candidates and medical staff as it is today.

We were walking on the brink. Within the jumble of words and terms, reprimands, and justifications, the organ shortage was the only solid fact. Even words such as "donation" and "altruism" had lost their meaning to me. I looked for a handle, something solid and clear to hold onto in the reality of my life and the lives of other people requiring kidney transplants. The shortage itself served as such a handle. Therefore, instead of mapping the political economy of organ transplants from an ideological and normative point of departure – in a utopian or dystopian discourse – it was the actual channels of organs from one body to another and their associated moral envelopes that served as my point of departure for understanding the grim reality I was in. This approach suspends the judgment that goes hand in hand with the issues surrounding organ transplants and expresses the view that is the shortage which is the basis upon which the organ moral economy grows and develops. This choice led me to a different understanding of the world of organ transplants than the one painted by ethicists, on the one hand, and anthropologists, on the other hand. I sought to tell a story that differed from the ethics and morals I found in the literature. I wanted to tell the story of the liminal zones, where categories blur. The transplant in Turkey taught me that the moral conceptualization of the movement of the organ from one body to another – from pure altruism to the raw utilitarianism embodied in the organ trade – depends on the sphere in which that movement occurs. This transplant taught me the experience of the lonely journey. It was lonely because contrary to the previous transplants and the one that would occur 16 years later, this transplant led me beyond the boundaries of the ethical and moral order. It was a journey that began with the oppressive realization that organ donations based a comprehensive sense of social solidarity, namely postmortem donations, fall well short of supplying the demand for transplant organs. I knew that another kind of donations – at the beginning of the journey I did not yet call it "the living organ economy" – depended on social and economic capital. They depend on family, social circles, personal connections, and work environment; most important of all is knowing other patients waiting for a transplant, who can lead the way to the organ dealers.

Waiting for a cadaveric donation is frustrating. On radio and television, we hear noble stories: the Arab who donated to a Jew and whose souls bonded, the family that decided to donate the organs of their dead child, and more and more moving stories of generosity, charity, and social solidarity. But at the dialysis clinic – sitting in armchairs, hooked up to the dialysis machines arranged in the shape of a U, 10 or 12 patients in each session of 3–5 hours – those stories seem far away. At the dialysis clinic, the realization dawns that looking for a kidney for transplant is, on the one hand, a completely personal matter and a hope shared by all. On the other hand, its realization depends on the social position and personal initiative of each one of us. A common fate that condemns us to seek a remedy alone.

The feeling of being caught in a no-man's land, an unmarked territory where you must navigate and find your way alone, with whatever means you have. That is the starting point where you must recalculate the relationship between morals and shortage. Then comes the politics of shortage: it is evident in what in the previous chapter, was called the "organ economy," and more specifically the organ economy of the household, the economy of the organ market, and the state's organ economy. My decision to go to the organ market involved deep mental anguish, but it is consistent with a general trend that will be detailed in the following chapters: a growing erosion of the formal organ economy, and transition from waiting for an organ, based on a broad concept of social solidarity, to active initiative to find a transplanted organ, based on privatization and individualization processes.

Therefore, the shortage shows the way in the dialysis clinics, in the long waiting hours in the lobbies of the nephrology clinics, and, of course, on the social networks. It is not a regular shortage economy, which is concerned with allocating resources in a state of shortage, but a strange informal economy that deals with human organs. It is a "shadow economy," which like the shadow cast by an illuminated object is cast by the formal economy. The organ trade is the extreme manifestation of the shadow economy.

The clear knowledge that there is no solution except the one we find for ourselves redraws the boundaries of the political, which is to say the boundaries of the possible. At that moment of realization, the shortage becomes a personal challenge. It is a moment of astonishment, followed by cynicism and irony, and, finally, awakening. At first, I was consumed by a sense of power, urgency, and desire to act. My main memory from that time is the loss of discretion. When solid ethical rules are cracked, broken, and crumbled, you know no limits. You could say that I switched to a "do it yourself" mode. I became my own medical case manager. I had my overt case as a transplant candidate, but meanwhile, I underwent classification and compatibility tests with potential sellers. All of the ethical questions – which in the formal economy belong to the category of "allocating organs for transplant" and are subject to considerations of which the patient's good is only one – became consumer questions. But the sense of power dissipated quickly and I learned that the rules of the game are set by the big profiteers, the traders. What I thought was possible turned out to be impossible, the political was revealed again not as the limits of the possible but its limitations.

In retrospect, after becoming acquainted with the world of the organ trafficking, I understand how lucky I was that I was not deceived and exploited and that the transplant was performed professionally. I am happy to say that the kidney seller also went through the operation successfully. I met him after the transplant, contrary to the recommendations I had received. "He's going to blackmail you," I was warned. For me, it wasn't even a question. We met at the clinic in Istanbul, and he told me he was newly divorced and the father of a baby girl. Three or four days later, he recovered and went back to Israel. When I got back to Israel, I contacted him. It turned out he had not made sure to do the necessary periodic tests. He covered the surgery scar with a large tattoo. He told me that his brother and other acquaintances of his who had sold their kidneys also covered their scars with tattoos so that no questions would be asked. The money that he and his brother received, he said, covered their debt to Social Security. He added that selling a kidney was a common solution in his neighborhood. He knew several people who had gone through it, and after they came back safe and sound, he and his brother decided to do it as well. The social distance between us was starkly evident, with no sublimation. His distress caused him to sell a kidney, whereas my distress caused me to buy a kidney. That action illustrated the connection between economy, health, and body, without the adornment of capitalist culture. It was like looking directly into the wound consuming the social body and seeing it at its ugliest.

The kidney sellers are quick to retreat back into their anonymity. My kidney seller remarried and moved to central Israel, and our relationship slackened. When I called him, he answered unwillingly and often didn't answer at all. Once I talked on the phone with his wife. I realized she did not know who I was and what I had to do with her husband, and she hurried to end the conversation. In 2008, when the transplant law and financial refunds to kidney donors were announced in Israel, he called me to ask if he was considered a kidney donor. I told him it only applied to future donors. Since then, our relationship was cut off completely. I devoted my doctoral thesis to him without giving his whole name. To this day, I shudder when I think of him. I asked him in Turkey: why sell a kidney of all things? "I need the money," he said, "but I'm also helping someone while I'm at it." The simplicity with which he bound his personal interest and helping an anonymous other was so contrary to the dichotomy between utilitarianism and altruism that it seemed as if all it would take was the lightest touch for the whole ethical construction of organ donations to collapse in front of my eyes.

I was very happy for my good luck, and that the kidney took and functions. However, I nurture a certain sense of shame. The moral dilemma continues to occupy me, but I know full well that the donation gave me life. My family, my children, my work, my daily routine – all were made possible by the transplant. Therefore, I live in a sort of constant sense of gratitude. It is a clear and simple feeling, arising from the knowledge that I am alive thanks to others – but also from a deeper understanding that needing the help of others accompanies every organ transplantee forever. Ultimately, the organ will be rejected and you will be sent out yet again into the stormy ocean of looking for a transplanted organ all over again. We are never a lonely island, as the poet John Donne wrote, we are part of humanity. Being an organ transplantee means understanding that poetic truth afresh in its modern, technological, but mostly human sense.

4   Global organ economy

Organ supply between the private and the public

The division of the organ economy into living organ economy and deceased organ economy largely overlaps with the division between the private sphere and the public sphere. The state channels deceased organs through public routes and operate formal mechanisms of organ procurement and allocation. The black market of trafficked organs operates in the shadows, far from the public eye, and the household organ economy conceals its donation dynamics under the cloak of privacy, often feigning a perfect donation relationship to obtain formal approval of the transplant.

The public–private distinction is crucial when examining the initiative to supply an organ. When the initiative comes from the patient or their family, the supply of organs is an act of the private sphere: it is the patient alone that embarks on a quest to find an organ and the respective potential donors come from the patient's social circles and social capital. When the initiative comes from the state, and the donation is facilitated by state mechanisms, the supply of organs can be viewed as an act of the public sphere.

This distinction will serve us here as the methodological point of departure of the analysis of the trends between public and private channels of organ supply. In the following pages, we will quantify these trends by examining the respective volumes of living organ economy out of the total organ economy in a given time and place. Estimating the trends of public and private sources of organ supply allows a more informed discussion on the changing ethics of organ donation. But first, in order to fully understand the distinction between private living organ economy and public organ economy, it is essential to contextualize organ economy as part of the political economy of health resources allocation.

The division of the welfare economy between private and public spheres is usually discussed in relation to the shrinking or expansion of public responsibility for social programs (Powell 2007). Privatization is, thus, understood as the transfer of responsibility over welfare to the hands of the individuals themselves and their families (Papadopoulos and Roumpakis 2019, Björnberg and Latta 2007). It is this sense of privatization – rather than the sale of public assets and welfare mechanisms to private entrepreneurs – which sits at the heart of the analysis offered

DOI: 10.4324/9781003288886-7

here. In that sense, privatization, or the interplay between private and public is not only a game limited to the market and state players. It is not the debate over which actor – free-market entrepreneurs or state bureaucrats – can reach better results. It is not even a normative discussion on who should bear responsibility for welfare – the citizen or the state. In this analysis, privatization refers to areas of welfare need that remain without institutional patronage or with limited and weak patronage. In these areas, where neither the state nor the market has the interest, ability, or permission to act, the family rises as the agent of welfare (Grootegoed and Van Dijk 2012).

The division between private and public spheres of activity is a dynamic division. The very concepts of "private" and "public" are constantly changing. Social institutions, organizations, and players move from one category to another. For example, if family members are paid public monies by the government for their care for their relative, is it an act in the private sphere? Conversely, if community members volunteer to help their needed neighbors – in what sense this pertains to the public sector of welfare economy?

In the context of transplant medicine, the plot further thickens. In a deceased organ economy, the organ is donated by the individual after their death, provided they expressed their consent to do so and the family gave its consent. This consent reflects a certain philosophy of the body after death: the body then loses its privacy and its organs move from the private domain to the public domain and are perceived as a sort of public or social goods, i.e., benefits all and free of pay (Oakland 1987). The decision as to the allocation of the donated organs is wholly given to the agents operating in the public domain. The donor's organs – neither the person, nor their whole body – are what is being donated to society at large. This is an important point because it emphasizes that the unit of analysis here is the organs themselves which can travel on different routes from one body to another and are charged respectively with different economic meanings. Interestingly, in deceased organ donation, the concept of self dies with the subject, but this death is not the death of the organs: those can travel to another body and in their travel are perceived as pertaining to the public. Deceased organ economy challenges the accepted division between private and public. The procurement of organs, by the formula of informed consent or presumed consent, emphasizes, on the one hand, the division between private and public, especially on the question of ownership of the body and the question of autonomy. Informed consent emphasizes the private-autonomous aspect of the donation, whereas presumed consent emphasizes its collective aspect. On the other hand, the consent transfers the organs of the cadaver all at once to a status of goods for distribution by standards decided by the health authorities. The transition from the private to the public is sharp. Having said that, it is important to note that in both cases – informed or presumed consent – the wishes of the dead do not supersede the wishes of the family: family opposition can undermine the donation even if the person expressed their explicit wish to donate their organs after death.

Living donations also pose a complicated challenge to the division between private and public. In living donations, the actual organ procurement is beyond the reach of the state or its agents. It is completely the result of private initiatives of patients and their families. The state is allowed to approve or disapprove the donation, but it cannot initiate it, asking even someone to volunteer and donate a kidney to someone else. However, the very approval or disapproval sets the fabric of relations between the living donor and the recipient in a predetermined moral pattern, which is presented as the appropriate pattern for that relationship. Organ supply is always an altruistic donation when it comes to state officials. The complicated and complex relationship that leads to the decision to donate an organ is thusly reduced to a rigid pattern subject to simplistic technocratic logic. For the donation to be approved, a close and ongoing relationship is required, but the motives for donation can be diverse, sometimes conflicting, and sometimes unconscious. Often the donation is the result of tacit agreement deriving from the very kinship, from the obviousness of the donation; often it is the result of coercion and force. Technocracy wishes to trap within the narrow confines of its moral default choices complicated and conflicted private mental worlds. In this case, the division between the private and the public blurs in the light of the state's power to approve or disapprove the donation, and in light of its ability to codify the world of interpersonal relationships according to an external moral logic, according to the altruistic code.

Thus, it appears that what was considered private (what motivated you to donate an organ to a relative or stranger) is encoded into an ethical language of normative narrative of donation and altruism. Meanwhile, the donated organs, once having become social goods, are distributed based on community boundaries. But, what are the social considerations of organ allocation? We saw in Chapter 1 that as soon as the first dialysis machines were operated in Seattle, it was proposed to limit entitlement to dialysis to citizens of Washington State whose taxes funded the experimental technology. What are the features of entitlement for organs when these are donated for the benefit of an anonymous patient? What are the physical boundaries of those entitled to this act of altruism? The city, the state, the region?

Health resources are often allocated by state health agencies to the citizens (and sometimes residents) of a given country. In more privatized system, health resources are provided according to insurance ownership. Deceased organs pertain to the model of the state as health providers. In some cases, transplant organizations are regional and range beyond the state borders (Eurotransplant, for example). In these cases, the reach of the public sphere of organ supply extends. The assumption, it seems, is that the altruistic donation grants an unlimited ethical space to channel the donated organ. If altruism stands for unconditional universal giving, then the donated organ can travel beyond the donor's own community, past the donor's national collective, and be transplanted into a patient according to regional agreements. This is not a criticism but another example of the transfer in the status and the ownership of the organ – a kidney, a liver, a heart, or any other organ – from the personal to the public.

The interplay between the private and the public in organ economies is fascinating. But from the standpoint of a patient in a need of an organ, this interplay frustrates you. I would rather prefer to receive an organ that was donated as an expression of solidarity and altruism from any of my fellow citizens. But, the shortage sadly indicates that such solidarity is lacking. Applying to private channels of organ supply, being in eternal debt of gratitude to a person you know, or even worse, paying someone for an organ – this is the actual face of privatization in organ economy.

At the global level, the distinction between the public and private is even more complex. Globalization processes have deepened the hold of organ markets beneath the reach of state authorities. On the other hand, the same processes have also led to the hegemony of the altruistic code and the brain death definition. Yet, the private–public distinction shapes in different local contexts in response to globalization.

A global organ economy

The first division of the global organ economy is according to the question of whether or not a given country provides transplantation services. In many countries, including those of central Africa, there is no transplantation medicine at all. South Africa is the only African country with a dual economy of living and deceased organ donations (Moosa 2019). Tunisia, Libya, Kenya, Sudan, Morocco, Algeria, Egypt, Nigeria, and Ghana are reported as having limited transplantation activity, exclusively based on living organ economy (Muller, White and Delmonico 2014). In central Africa, there is fierce resistance by public opinion leaders to organ transplantation, in general, and organs from the deceased, in particular. In North Africa, there is transplantation medicine based mainly on living organs. In Egypt, for instance, kidney transplantations are performed only by living donors. Even after the Egyptian parliament approved the brain death law in 2010, no transplants were performed on the deceased as a result of religious disputes over the definition of brain death (Hamdy 2012). Generally, in many parts of Africa, transplantation medicine is sideswept by more urgent challenges: malnutrition, infectious diseases, and fear of epidemic outbreaks (Naicker 2009). In some countries in Central Asia (such as Afghanistan and Turkmenistan), there is no transplantation medicine at all or it is undeveloped (Ghods 2015, Budiani 2007).

But, transplantation medicine has spread throughout the world in considerable volume. In order to examine organ economies and trace the interaction between the deceased organ economy and the living organ economy in countries that operate transplantation medicine, it is necessary to discern between different variants of organ economy in a given country. For a deceased organ economy to exist, a given county must have an elaborated organizational infrastructure for the procurement and allotment of organs based on waiting lists for performing the maximum matching between the donor and the recipient in a short time interval and with no advance preparation, which requires an extensive array of data sets and laboratories. As noted earlier, a deceased organ economy also requires, given the dead donor rule, consensus over the definition of brain death. Even if that definition is anchored in legislation or internal regulations, consensus over it must be broad; to achieve agreement to donate an organ from the deceased, the definition of brain death must exceed professional circles and be accepted by the public. The Japanese, Israeli, and many other cases, for instance, indicate that even with a brain death law an agreed medical protocol to define brain death, public resistance to the definition of brain death can be an obstacle for the deceased organ economy even in countries with extensive health infrastructures and high medical and technological capabilities.

To examine the organ economy from a global perspective, I borrow Emmanuel Wallerstein's model of global dispositions of core, periphery, and semi-periphery regions in the world system (Wallerstein 2004). Wallerstein's theory can help us draw the outline of the global order of organ economy. According to Wallerstein, the world economic system is made of three concentric circles: the core areas circle, the semi-periphery circle, and the periphery circle. When it comes to the organ economy, the core areas include the countries that have the medical infrastructure to perform organ transplantations and provide long-term care to the transplanted. These countries also have the organizational and systemic infrastructure for the existence of a deceased organ economy, and there is a mechanism designated for the cultivation of such an economy, namely, public education campaigns to encourage organ donation. In the core countries, the procurement and allocation of organs follow laws and rules accommodated to the voluntary donation model, and allocation is based on insurance entitlement and medical priority. In other words, in the core countries, the formal organ economy is an option the state provides to those who need transplants. Evidently, the core countries of organ economy are usually also the core countries of the world system, i.e., are concentrated in Europe and North America.

In the semi-periphery countries – Saudi Arabia, for example – there is a suitable medical array for performing transplantations from the deceased, and the treatment and follow-up of transplantees, and there are also organizational infrastructures and regulation systems – through laws or regulations – to procure organs from the deceased. But unlike the core countries, the semi-periphery countries do not manage to develop a sufficient deceased organ economy because of the scarcity of postmortem organ donations. This is evidenced by the long lines for transplants in these countries, with waiting time for organs, sometimes, extending to the point of futility.

To be sure, in the core countries, there is also a chronic and ongoing shortage of organs, and in them too, the organ economy is a shortage economy. But, the difference is in how the shortage problem is confronted. In the core countries, the existence of a developed deceased organ economy mitigates the shortage problem within the formal sector of the organ economy and its severity is several levels less than in the periphery or semi-periphery countries. Conversely, in the periphery and semi-periphery countries, the shortage problem is mainly confronted by a living organ economy.

The periphery countries are countries that have the suitable medical technology and operate transplantation centers but lack all the other components of an organ economy. In these countries, the organ economy relies on living organs, without regulation and without tight control of the source of the transplantation organs. Furthermore, the health challenges in these countries are twofold, which adds an even greater burden for numerous countries, especially in Asia and Africa: along with treating chronic conditions, such as kidney failure or lung, heart, and liver disease, they also deal with the danger of infectious disease outbreaks. Moreover, the adaptation of the Western lifestyle and diet increases the spread of chronic disease such as diabetes and hypertension (Boutayeb 2010). These diseases can lead to failures whose best solution is transplantation. The growing demand for organ transplantation, coupled with an insufficient organizational infrastructure, makes the organ shortage in the peripheral regions especially acute. Furthermore, sometimes, the citizens of those countries are not entitled to transplantation surgery as part of the local health system, and their transplantation centers serve mainly patients from abroad in a model that skirts closely if not actually crossing the line to organ trafficking. An example of a peripheral state is Indonesia. Since the beginning of its transplantation medicine, in the late 1970s, only a few hundred kidney transplants have been performed in Indonesia. That is a negligible number, particularly considering the country's population of hundreds of millions. In 2013, the brain death law was passed in Indonesia, but since then, only one single transplantation was performed there from a deceased donor.

In each one of the circles, core, semi-periphery, and periphery, there is also an internal division. Spain and Italy, for instance, are clear core countries based on the standards described above. The United States is also a core country, but as we shall see below, the ways it deals with the shortage problem are different, and it has a thriving living organ economy, much more than the living organ economy in Spain and Italy. These differences can be attributed to the different constellations of the private–public distinction in health policies and their impact on the role of private initiatives of organ supply.

The classification between core, periphery, and semi-periphery corresponds with different modes of local political economy of public and private channels of organ supply. Whereas in peripheral organ economy, a public sector of organ economy simply does not exist, in core and semi-peripheral organ economy, the distinction between public and private plays a central role in what is understood here as privatization. Such a process cannot take place without the presence of two sectors. In the absence of a public sector, such as in peripheral organ economies, organ economy is sparse and thin and is composed of living individuals whose motives cannot be confirmed.

Moreover, the classification of these three circles is not rigid and there is mobility between them, especially between the core circle and the semi-periphery circle. So, for example, Brazil has managed, in recent years, to establish a deceased organ economy and can be said to have moved from the semi-periphery to the core circle. On the other hand, Tunisia was the only North African country that had a deceased organ economy (albeit small). After the 2010 revolution, which ushered in the Arab Spring, its organ donations dropped sharply and it was pushed into the periphery circle. Likewise, the spread of transplantation medicine throughout the world expanded the periphery circle. The countries of Central Asia, for instance, began to perform organ transplants – albeit on a minute scale – at the beginning of the 2010s. Again, organ economies in the periphery circle are characterized by ongoing and permanent reliance on living organs, and Egypt is a good example of that effect.

The shortage is what motivates the organ economy. Each circle has a differing degree of shortage, but the shortage can clearly be rated as very severe in the periphery countries, severe in the semi-periphery countries, and serious in the core countries. The difference is in how the shortage problem is confronted. In the core countries, the existence of a deceased organ economy merges the shortage problem into the formal organ economy sector.

The division into core, semi-periphery, and periphery countries allows to extract ourselves from the binary distinction between altruistic donation and organ trafficking. In fact, characteristics of altruistic donation, on the one hand, and trafficking, on the other hand, can be found in each one of the three circles of the global organ economy: a living organ economy does not necessarily indicate organ trafficking and a deceased organ economy does not necessarily indicate pure altruism, but rather more effective procurement mechanisms. Organ economies operate within a particular geopolitical context; they are embedded in a social–political fabric that changes along with the global political economy. Therefore, the severity of the shortage and availability of transplantation medicine depends not only on local factors – including the existence of a transplantation system and infrastructure for the procurement of deceased organs, consensus over the definition of brain death, and trust in the medical system – but also on geopolitical position within the global neoliberal order.

The privatization of organ economy

The global order of the organ economy can be characterized by the degree of institutionalization of the deceased organ economy in a certain country at a certain time. There is an organ shortage in the whole world, but waiting lists to receive an organ from a deceased donor differ in length: the wait for an organ in Sweden is different from the wait for an organ in Singapore or Cyprus, for example. Surely, this is true for other limited healthcare resources. The global distribution of vaccines to COVID-19 during the pandemic is a recent example of a global scale unequal distribution of health resources. As a matter of fact, the organ shortage gets lost in the general shortage of healthcare resources. The lack of medications, hospital beds, life support machines, and other health resources is far more too severe as it impacts the health of millions around the world.

But the shortage of organs is unique in the ways patients in need find in order to cope with it. As we have seen, the source of organs for transplantation is two-fold: from the living and from the dead. And the supply basis is threefold: state, family, and market. This structure creates a range of options of obtaining an organ outside the formal channels. For instance, organ donation within the family is considered legitimate and can alleviate the shortage without using the state's limited pool of organs for transplantations and without going underground and illegally buying an organ.

In areas where the organ shortage is particularly severe, with waiting times for organs measured in years and sometimes being futile, the transition of kidney patients to personally searching for an organ is undertaken directly and straight-forwardly. Patients simply do not wait to be registered for a deceased donation and come up – in different ways – with their living donor. In places where transplant units work without a supportive institutional array of national transplant centers or transplant coordinators, an organ economy emerges that is totally mediated in the private sphere. Unlike organ transplantation from the dead, the search for an organ from the living does not require formal registration, and for kidney patients, this search can begin even before one enters into dialysis treatments which is – in many places – the benchmark for entering formal waiting lists for a deceased kidney donation. In families that know they have a genetic disease that harms the kidneys, whether or not family members are carriers of the gene that causes the disease is what will determine who will be the potential donors and who the potential recipients.

Since the subject of this book is the political economy of transplantation organs, the emphasis here is on ways of procuring organs and on the social institutions that participate in the procurement and allocation of organs for transplantation. Therefore, it is important to actually distinguish between the ordered and bureau-cratic structure of the deceased organ economy, and the open, network structure of the living organ economy as a household economy or black market. The dis-tinction between the deceased organ economy and the living organ economy is of methodological importance. It refers to private vs. public organ procurement mechanisms. The living organ economy usually belongs to the informal organ economy. Therefore, the rate of living donations out of the total organ donations may testify, albeit partially, to the volume of the privatization process, the extent to which organs are sought by the patient and their family and are not supplied by the state.

The privatization in organ economy refers to the transfer of providing an organ for transplantation from the state to the patient. At the backdrop of an exac-erbating shortage in deceased organ donations, more and more patient embark on a personal quest to find themselves their life-saving organ. Where the state is involved in initiating a deceased organ donation (through presumed consent models and by transplant coordinators in ICU's), it cannot be involved in initi-ating a living organ donation. It cannot ask H to donate her kidney to M. This can only come from the free, self-determined, and autonomous will of H herself. Therefore, rates of living organ donation – or the extent of living organ economy in the terms of this book – tell the story of organ economy's privatization trends.

Organ donations from living people are registered in transplantation organiza-tion databases all over the world. These databases lack data that could have pro-vided a fuller picture of this privatization process, especially of the black market, for instance, the number of transplantees whose transplants were not reported, or the number of patients who did not undergo a donation approval process but underwent transplantations in unknown locations. Nonetheless, those records can indicate, if only by negation, the relative power of the formal and informal organ procurement mechanisms. Data published by transplantation organizations might, therefore, help examine the ratio between the use of organs from living donors and the use of organs from deceased donors over time in a given country.

The data I use was taken from the records of the Spanish center TPM–DTI Transplant Donation – Management Procurement Transplant Institute located in Barcelona.[1] The center collects official data from transplantation organizations in more than 90 countries around the world since 1998. Its database is open to the public. Not all countries have provided consistent and full information over the years and much data is lacking, especially about periphery countries. This database distinguishes between organ donations by source of donation (living or deceased) and organ. This distinction helps understand the fluctuations in the organ economy because it allows to add up the donations from the living and the dead for a total of organ donations in a certain country in a certain year. The focus is on actual donations rather than transplantations because while a living donation leads to the transplantation of a single organ (usually a kidney), donations from the deceased lead to more transplantations (sometimes up to seven organs). So that the comparison between transplantations performed with organs taken from the deceased can tilt the picture and appear as if there are much more organ donations from the families of people who consented to donate their organs after their death, but this is not the case. The center notes donations of organs from the deceased and in a separate column organ donations from the deceased after cardiac death (that is, not after brain death).

The calculation of the rate of the living organ economy out of the total organ economy was made in the following way: First, the volume of the deceased organ economy was calculated as the total deceased donations and deceased donations after cardiac death. Then, the total of organ donations was calculated as organ donations from living people plus deceased donations. The rate of the living organ donations was calculated by dividing the living organ donations from the total organ economy in a certain country in a certain year. All of the data was weighted per million people (p.m.p.). Taking living organ economy as a proxy of privatized ways of obtaining organs, that is searching for an organ without the help of state or other formal agencies, high percentages indicate high levels of privatization in a given country in a given time.

Four cases of organ economies

The table below shows the rate of living organ donations out of total organ donations in the 20 years between 2000 and 2019 in four selected countries: two core countries (the United Kingdom and Spain) and two semi-periphery countries, one of which became a core country (Brazil) and another (Saudi Arabia) with a dominant living organ economy. In the following pages, I will detail the dynamics of the organ economy in each one of the four countries for a closer look on interplay between the local and the global in organ economy.

Table 4.1 Percentages of living donations out of total organ donations in four countries: 2000–2019

Year	UK	Spain (%)	Brazil (%)	Saudi Arabia (%)
2000	31	1	72	84
2001	31	4	73	80
2002	31	5	66	86
2003	37	6	63	83
2004	34	5	59	78
2005	38	6	65	77
2006	42	7	64	66
2007	45	9	61	75
2008	45	10	59	72
2009	44	13	52	81
2010	51	15	49	80
2011	42	17	46	86
2012	39	18	40	88
2013	38	18	37	91
2014	39	21	36	86
2015	38	15	33	90
2016	34	10	31	90
2017	33	11	25	89
2018	32	9	25	90
2019	31	10	25	91

The United Kingdom

The British National Health System (NHS) is a public and universal health system mostly funded by taxes (Cylus, Richardson, Findley et al. 2015). In each one of the four countries that comprise the United Kingdom – Northern Ireland, Scotland, Wales, and England – there is a separate healthcare system, and the procurement and allocation of transplantation organs are undertaken within the framework of the state under various laws and regulations. In all of the countries that comprise the United Kingdom, organ transplantation is part of general insurance coverage. In international analyses of fluctuations in organ donations, the UK system is viewed as a single system. The British organ economy has an interesting story over the last 20 years. In 2000, the volume of the living organ economy out of the total organ economy was 31%, and the same was true 20 years later in 2019. But over those years, the number of organ donations from the living rose, and in 2010, exactly halfway through the time period, there were more donations from living people than donations harvested from the deceased. The first decade of the century was on a rising trajectory of organ donations from the living, whereas the second decade was on a dropping trajectory down to the opening point of the millennium.

The second decade of the century was relatively turbulent. During the decade, there were numerous discussions of the method of organ harvesting from the dead and the opt-in model enacted in the United Kingdom was replaced in 2020 by "presumed consent," after the same change was made in Scotland in 2019 and in Wales in 2015. There is not enough data yet to assess the impact of the legal change on patterns in the organ economy and whether the change will lead to an increase in organ donations from the deceased and a reduction in the living organ economy. Studies do indicate that the policy change has led to an increase in the deceased organ economy, but at least one study of the differences between countries that adopt the opt-in model and countries that adopt the presumed consent model found that the transition to presumed consent has a negative effect on the number of donations from living donors (Arshad, Anderson and Sharif 2019). This is an interesting finding because it raises the possibility that such a transition, contrary to the intentions, does not necessarily lead to an increase in the pool of transplantation organs but might even reduce it because of the drop in living donors.

According to the data shown here, the United Kingdom still has a dual organ economy that accounts for between 30% and 50% of total organ donations. The United Kingdom, like other core countries in the global organ economy, tries to increase the supply of both sources of organs – both from the deceased and donations from living people. We must remember in this context that increasing the supply of organs from the deceased benefits all who need transplants, namely those who are in need of a donation from the deceased, who are waiting for heart, lung, liver, and pancreas transplants. The effort to increase the volume of donations from the deceased leads to searching for additional sources of deceased organs besides those who have undergone brain death. More and more organ donations in the United Kingdom come from people who died cardiac death. In 2000, such donations were relatively rare and only 38 donations came from donors after cardiac death. Twenty years later, the number of donations after cardiac death was 689. A 16-fold increase. Post-cardiac death donation is a good solution for donation, considering that the definition of brain death is not broadly accepted and it enables approaching and gaining consent even from families that oppose the definition of brain death. The existence of a post-cardiac death organ donation system can be an indication of an organ procurement system that is culturally competent and sufficiently technologically and logistically developed to overcome the blood insufficiency to the organs after cardiac death and performs successful transplants even from that source.

Therefore, it is interesting to note that alongside the effort to increase the volume of the deceased organ economy, the British National Health System Blood and Transplant NHSBT also set itself the goal of increasing the volume of the living organ economy. In a strategic document issued in 2014, the organization listed the advantages of organ transplants from living donors, including better clinical results, planning transplantation before dialysis, cost–benefit calculations of transplantation versus dialysis, and more.[2] The report found that compared to Wales, Scotland, and England, Northern Ireland had the highest rate of organ donations from the living. The document points to March 2020 as the goal when the rate of living donations would reach 26 donations per million. According to the 2019 data, the rate of living donors was far from that goal, reaching only 15.1 per million people.

In an updated document from 2017, the NHSBT specified that 97% of the donations were kidneys and 3% were liver lobes.[3] The living organ economy in Britain is organized by the United Kingdom Living Kidney Sharing System (UKLKSS), an NHS apparatus operating since 2012, which is the most developed in Europe in matching living kidney donors with recipients. The program sees to pair donations by crosschecks, donation chains that begin with an anonymous donor, applying ethical codes of donation without reward or stipulation, encouraging living donations, and more.

The British example is an interesting case of a core country working to promote both sectors of the organ economy – both from the living and from the dead. The British attempt is to exhaust the donation potential from every source while maintaining the accepted ethical rules of anonymous and unconditional donation. The transition to a presumed consent policy might increase the scope of deceased donations, but it should be hoped that such an increase does not lead to stagnation or decrease in the living organ economy that is regulated and managed through the UKLKSS. As we shall see below, the distribution of living donations through state mechanisms while maintaining the ethical rules of anonymity and unconditionality cannot always be taken for granted.

Spain

The Spanish healthcare system is universal and covers more than 99% of the population. The system is mostly funded by general taxation but private expenditures on health rose in the last decade and are higher than the average in other European countries. Life expectancy in Spain is the highest in Europe.[4] Spain is a world model of organ procurement and allocation policy. It has the highest rate of deceased organ donation in the world. According to the worldwide data collected for this study, Spain manages to increase the number of organ donations from the deceased every year. In 2019, the rate of donations from the deceased was nearly 66 donations per million people. For comparison, in the same year in the United States, the rate of donations from the deceased was only 44 per million people. Furthermore, Spain is also perceived as an organizational success story, and the "Spanish model" for organ donation procurement has long become the "golden rule," and standard for how to obtain consent for donation from the families of the deceased. This model grants utmost importance to the transplant coordinators in the hospitals and their professional training. Usually, these coordinators are nurses trained specifically for that mission with an expertise of approaching families in their most distressing moments and asking for an organ donation.

Furthermore, Spain has a "presumed consent" model for organ donation, and the prevailing Catholic faith may also help promote donations, seen as an act of grace. In fact, for Catholics, organ donation does not pose a difficulty, neither as far as the definition of brain death nor concerning questions about the integrity of the body or resurrection, like in other faiths. It is even possible that the Catholic emphasis on the redemption of the soul, and the sacrifice of Jesus's body, may even help promote the cultural and normative acceptance of postmortem organ donation. Evidence may be seen in the high rates of postmortem organ donation in Italy and Ireland as well. In Spain too, like in the United Kingdom, along with post-brain death organ donations, there has also been a sharp rise in the last 20 years in organ donation after cardiac death. In 2000, the number of such cases was slightly above 30. Twenty years, later the number of cases reached 745, almost a quarter of total post-mortem organ donations.

Yet, the data in the table above indicates a rise of the living organ economy in Spain as well, perhaps the most quintessential core state in the global organ economy. While in 2000, only 1% of the total organ economy was of donations from living people, during the studied period, the rate of the living organ economy rose considerably, reaching more than 20% by 2014. The rise in the living organ economy, like the rise in the United Kingdom, is the result of a deliberate effort by the organ transplant procurement organizations. Like in Britain, the reliance on organ donations from the deceased, even in light of Spain's successful record, is not enough. Thus, the successful effort to increase the use of post-cardiac death organ donations, as well as drafting a dedicated program to expand the base of living donors.

This program has been operating in Spain since 2005. Valentin et al. (2018) report that organ donation from the living is encouraged through public campaigns to raise awareness of living donations, crosscheck programs, protocols for procuring donations from strangers, and their allocation with the Spanish transplant center(ONT), which operates a registration mechanism for living donors similar to the British UKLKSS.

Both Spain and the United Kingdom are examples of core countries in the global economy of transplantation organs. In both countries, we see a rise in the volume of organ donations in the studied period. In Spain, the total number of donations, in 2000, was 1,396 (including only 19 from living donors), whereas in 2020, the total number of donations reached 3,382 (of which 335 were from living donors) – an almost 2.5-fold rise. In the United Kingdom, the organ economy grew over that 20-year period almost threefold. Those expansions, unlike organ economies in semi-periphery and periphery areas as we shall see, are the outcome of an increase in the organ pool from both living and deceased people combined. That expansion is the result of a designed effort and implementation of dedicated programs to procure organ donations from both sources: both the living and the dead.

Whereas expansion of the organ procurement mechanisms from the dead is a refinement of existing procurement mechanisms that characterize, as we have seen in the previous chapter, the monopoly of the state and its agencies over the deceased organ economy, the models to expand the circle of living organ donors indicate an interesting variant of the political economy of transplantation organs in the core countries. These programs offer a combination between the private and public spheres of the organ economy. After all, donations from living people are always a personal initiative that resides fully in the private sphere. As aforementioned, the state cannot compel John to donate to Jane. But once the desire to donate appears, the question of the regulation of the donation itself, its examination, and its approval or disapproval for different reasons move into the purview of the public sphere. The advantage of incorporating an allocation system of living donor organs, such as the British UKLKSS, is that it promises that those donations will not create a discriminatory system that stipulates donations on arbitrary criteria and that the organ will reach the patient who needs it the most. In other words, the main role of national programs to encourage living donations is to create sharing, namely, a sharing of the donations between the donors and those who need them, by turning the altruistic motive into a mechanism of solidarity. As we shall see, control of the allocation mechanism of living donations is not always as absolute as in the Spanish and British examples and other core countries.

Brazil

The Brazilian healthcare system is a decentralized system that operates on three levels: federal, state, and local. The right to health is granted by the Brazilian Constitution and is imparted to all residents of Brazil free of charge and freely through the Unified Health System (SUS).[5] Among the BRICS countries, Brazil has the broadest and most comprehensive public healthcare system. The decentralization between three administrative levels creates gaps in access to healthcare between different parts of the population, between and within Brazilian states. However, international indexes indicate a constant improvement in the general healthcare coverage of the population.[6] Brazil is in the second place worldwide in the absolute number of organ transplants it performs (after the United States). The Brazilian transplantation law from 1997 caused a major uproar because of the policy of presumed consent to donation, and it was changed to informed consent in 2001. The Brazilian Ministry of Health outlines the transplantation policy, and the transplants are administered on the local level in coordination with the SUS. More than 95% of transplants in Brazil are funded by the public healthcare system and the rest privately.

In the early 2000s, its organ economy was mostly based on living organs (72%), but gradually, a deceased organ economy developed so that by 2017 only one-quarter of transplantation organs in Brazil were from living people. A study of the transplantation system in Brazil in 2017 found a significant increase in the number of transplantations that were performed, especially from deceased donors. However, it was also found that the expansion of the organ transplantation system developed mainly in the southern and southeastern Brazilian states, causing wide gaps in access to transplants. The researchers indicate the lack of a sufficient infrastructure for transplantations and dialysis in the northern Brazilian states, to the point that some of them record no dialysis patients. The researchers emphasize that access to transplants in Brazil is highly dependent on the patients' social background, especially an income that allows them to live near transplantation centers.[7]

The expansion of the transplantation system in the studied period is the result of the opening of transplantation centers and a deliberate effort by the SUS.

Most of the organ transplants are performed in Brazil's southern and southeastern states, where there has also been the most significant increase in organ donations between 2011 and 2017, and where the most suitable and fullest infrastructure for performing transplants is located (Gómez, Jungmann and Lima 2018).

This process is parallel to the general strengthening of the Brazilian public healthcare system in making healthcare services accessible to the population. Organ transplants are part of the general healthcare insurance coverage for residents of Brazil, and in terms formulated in this book, it can be stated that this process indicates Brazil's organ economy moving toward the circle of core countries. However, as noted above, studies indicate a clear distinction between north and south in transplants in Brazil. Transplantation medicine is much more developed in the south than in the north, and gaps between states in access to transplants are wide. This division may indicate an uncompleted process of improving transplantation medicine in Brazil. According to the data in the table, the process is moving in a positive direction. In the past decades, a transplantation medicine based on postmortem donations has developed in Brazil although not in the entire country, yet an efficient infrastructure for transplantations from the deceased has been erected in the southern states. It can be hoped that the Brazilian system will manage to expand its successful transplantation medicine to the northern countries as well.

Saudi Arabia

This country has a developed healthcare infrastructure funded by the state. About 80% of the healthcare services in the country are provided by the national healthcare system or its extensions to the residents of the kingdom (Almalki, Fitzgerald and Clark 2011). The first kidney transplant was performed in Saudi Arabia in 1979, and its national transplantation center opened in 1985. Saudi transplantation medicine does not lag behind Western countries in its transplant surgery, which had already performed hundreds of heart transplants and 285 lung transplants by 2017. The Saudi National Transplantation Center also publishes a peer-reviewed scientific journal, Saudi Journal of Kidney Diseases and Transplantations, which comes out six times a year. Furthermore, Saudi Arabia has an organ donation sharing system with the Gulf Cooperation Council (GCC) countries, which besides Saudi Arabia include the Gulf countries of Kuwait, Qatar, the United Arab Emirates, Oman, and Bahrain. Such regional cooperation also occurs in other places in the world. Since the organ exchange program between the countries was established in 1996, until 2019, Saudi Arabia had received 438 transplantation organs from its neighbors (Al-Attar 2020).

The attitude of the Sunni Islam that rules Saudi Arabia to organ transplantation is positive, and in a series of fatwas, the principle of brain death that allows organ transplantation from the dead was accepted (Albar 2012). Efforts to increase the trend of donations from the dead succeeded in the first decade of the 2000s (Shaheen, Al-Attar, Follero and Kamal 2017), but as the table above indicates, that trend slackened and the Saudi organ economy is still predominantly based on a living organ economy. Despite the means to diagnose cases of brain death in the emergency rooms, only 36% of the approaches to families elicited donations in 2019, producing 113 deceased donations (Al-Attar 2020a). On the other hand, 981 kidneys were transplanted that year from living donors, of which 875 kidneys came from the patients' relatives and 106 from living donors outside the family circles. It is worth noting that liver transplants as well in Saudi Arabia in 2019 relied more on the living organ economy: 241 transplants of liver lobes were performed from live donors compared to 78 livers donated from the deceased (Al-Attar 2020a).

Numerous studies have been made of the Saudi population's perceptions and approaches toward organ donation. The common findings between these studies indicate a relatively high level of knowledge about organ donations, but a lower level of approval of organ donation as per the official Sunni position, and aversion to postmortem donation, out of fear of violation and mutilation of the body after extracting the organs. The studies usually conclude that awareness of postmortem organ donation among the Saudi population should be raised (Alghanim 2010, Alam 2007).

But for the majority of organ donations in Saudi Arabia – the household economy upon which almost the entire organ economy in the country depends – there is no in-depth research. Data is lacking about the ratio between men and women donors, the kind of family relationship between donors and recipients, the ratio between men and women recipients, age, income, and more. We learn from other sources about the status of Saudi women in the strict patriarchal kingdom, which also impacts their health and access to healthcare services (Mobaraki and Soderfeldt 2010). Does the constitutional vulnerability of Saudi women also make them more vulnerable targets for organ donation? Is there a screening protocol for living donors in Saudi Arabia and what is it? Does it resemble the existing evaluation committees in different places in the world, and are there donor's advocates in Saudi Arabia? What is the nature of the relationship between unrelated donors and recipients?

The gray area of the living organ economy in Saudi Arabia positions it, according to the Wallersteinian model presented above, as a clear semi-periphery country: It has an elaborate infrastructure for transplantation medicine, including a scientific medical community, an organ exchange program with neighboring countries, and public information efforts to integrate the concept of brain death into the population and raise awareness of organ donation in general. Yet, at the same time, the Saudi organ economy is predominantly a living organ economy, and as such, it may also hide an organ supply involving power relations, especially gender power relations. In 2019, more than 20,000 Saudis were in dialysis treatment and waiting for a kidney donation (Al-Attar 2020). The shortage of organs for transplantation, especially those supplied through the deceased organ economy (113 donations that year), leads many patients to turn to the private channel of searching for an organ through relatives. But what is the cost of that channel?

The rise of living organ economy

A review of the trends in these four countries shows a complex picture of the distribution of labor between the private and the public, between the formal pro-curement mechanisms the state operates and through which it channels the de-ceased organ economy, and the constant presence of the living organ economy. An examination of the data in additional countries indicates a clear picture of the dual organ economy in core countries and the rise in living organ economy in semi-peripheral ones. The figure below illustrates this clearly in relation to six selected countries.

Thus, for instance, in Italy in 2000, 10% of the organ economy was comprised of a living organ economy, compared to 23% in 2019. In Germany, the volume of the living organ economy reached a record 48% in 2013. The trend has since dropped, and in 2019, the rate of the living organ economy was 38% of the total organ economy. In France too, living organ economy doubled (from 12% to 24%) during the first two decades of the century. France, Italy, and Germany, as well as Spain and the United Kingdom, are clear core countries both in the political economy of organ transplants and in the global political economy. The United States, however, presents an interesting case: whereas the European countries show transition from an economy predominantly reliant on a deceased organ economy, in the United States, the organ economy was a dual economy through-out the years. In 2000, half of the organ donations in the United States came from a living organ economy and that rate continued more or less through the first

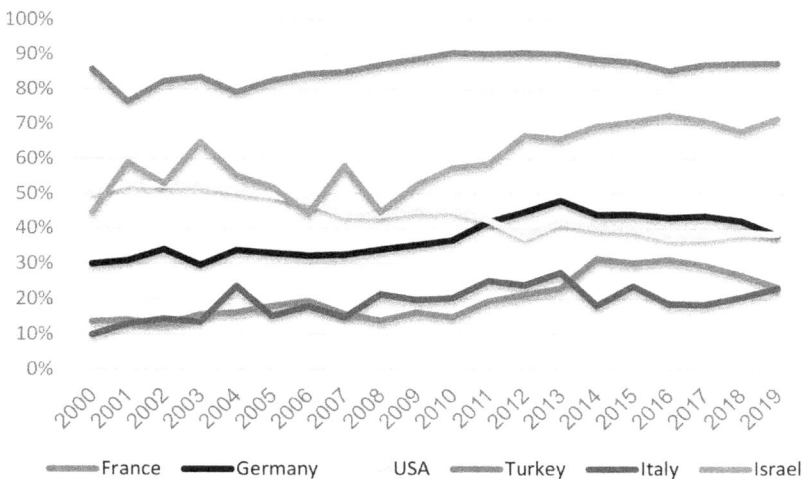

Figure 4.1 Percentages of living donations out of total organ donations in five countries: 2000–2019

Source: https://www.irodat.org/

decade of the century. The trend changed in the second decade and the volume of the deceased organ economy rose until in 2019 it reached 62%.[8]

The data from those countries indicate a rise in the general volume of organ procurement, including from the dead, but the rise in donations from the living indicates attempts to circumvent the state's official procurement and allocation mechanisms in favor of private channels of finding an organ for transplantation.

Two main points arise from the international data: first, the global organ economy is a dual economy. The ratio between the public sector of procuring donations from the dead and generating a deceased organ economy and the private sector that procures donations from living people changes from country to country and over time, but despite all of those changes, one cannot ignore the fact that the living organ economy functions as a central source of organ donations even in the core countries. In semi-periphery and periphery countries, the existence of a living organ economy is even more present. In many of those countries, most of the transplants come from living donors. Saudi Arabia is a good illustration, but Israel or Turkey, for instance, as we shall see below, are also cases in which the vast majority of the organ economy is based on a living organ economy. Is the existence of a living organ economy a vote of nonconfidence in the state's procurement and distribution mechanisms? Is it evidence of a worsening of the state of shortage? Increasing the volume of the organ economy as a whole indicates the development and expansion of transplantation medicine, in general, but that expansion puts an even greater spotlight on the shortage problem. Whereas the increase in the living organ economy indicates the path for many waiting for kidney transplants to receive the lifesaving organ. Furthermore, we must remember that the data that served to indicate the trend of the organ economy includes legal organ donations mainly of friends and family. The organ supply through the organ markets is not included in the statistics. Numerous patients travel to foreign countries to purchase organs on the black market and those transactions are not recorded at all.

At this point of the analysis, we can already indicate a main direction of movement in the political economy of organ transplants. That economy is based mainly on the desperate need to find an organ for transplantation outside of the formal waiting list. It is a lonely quest in the sense that it uses underground means. As aforesaid, the family is the main social institution in the legal living organ economy, but the search for a transplantation organ can exceed the family framework and occur on social networks established for that purpose. Therefore, the living organ economy relies on the family, social networks, and social capital. This economy is characterized by local patterns of organ procurement and consent for donation, which are not always consistent with the existing ethical guidelines in the public sphere of the formal organ economy. In the next chapter, I will elaborate on the growing gulf between the ethics that accompany the living organ economy and those that envelop the deceased organ economy, but a global organ economy is not only the sum of the country-based economies at a given time but also of regional organ exchange arrangements between countries, on the one hand, and the global organ trading networks, on the other hand. Moreover, the globalization processes are what enable the normative institutionalization of the voluntary donation code as the exclusive code for organ donation.

Beneath and above the state: market–state relations in the global organ economy

Turkey is a good place to begin a discussion of the globalization of organ transplantation. According to the terms that guide us in this chapter, Turkey is a semi-periphery country. It is a country with one of the highest rates of living organ economy even though it has the infrastructure for a deceased organ economy and established a transplantation coordination center in 2006 to encourage donations from the deceased. Yet, the consent rate for postmortem donations is low despite the Islamic permission to accept the definition of brain death. The rate of the living organ economy in Turkey, like Saudi Arabia, is around 90% and it is the European country with the highest rate of living donations.

In the Turkish case, it is not clear what the sociological breakdown of living donors is. Nor could I find credible documentation of a breakdown of the living donors between those donating to family members or to strangers. Nor did I find a clear protocol for the oversight of that kind of donation. In fact, as we shall see in the following chapters, Turkey was considered for years one of the main destinations of organ trafficking (Scheper-Hughes 2005). As told earlier in the biographical section "Istanbul 2004," I underwent my third transplant in that framework. In the first decade of the 21st century, according to Sanal (2004), most of the donations from living donors involved payment to the donor.

It is ironic that it was none other than Turkey that issued the most significant battle cry against organ trafficking. The Declaration of Istanbul is the most significant international effort to stop global trafficking in the country. In April 2008, the Transplantation Society (TTS) and the International Society of Nephrology (ISN) convened a summit meeting in Istanbul with more than 150 representatives from scientific and medical bodies, ethicists, sociologists, and government officials, who formulated the following treaties:

> The Declaration thus complements efforts by professional societies, national health authorities, and inter-governmental organizations such as the World Health Organization, the United Nations, and the Council of Europe to support the development of ethical programs for organ donation and transplantation, and to prevent organ trafficking and transplant tourism.[9]

The declaration actually recognizes the global difference between countries – which in the terms of this work are based solely on a living organ economy and countries based on a deceased organ economy, and which have the infrastructure and information systems to raise awareness of donations from the deceased. One of the goals of the declaration is to establish the supporting care of donors based on protocols that govern an organ donation screening process from living donors based on medical and psychosocial criteria, with an emphasis on informed consent as well as the welfare and health of the donor post-transplantation. The authors of the declaration consider it a continuation of the Universal Declaration of Human Rights from 1948 and thereby emphasize the universal nature of the declaration's values. Therefore, the fight against organ trafficking is part of the fight to create a just and equal world with equity in the universal right of every person to welfare and health.

A decade later, in 2018, the declaration was updated after a round of research and discussion to emphasize the importance of self-sufficiency and maximizing the potential of organ donations from the deceased in each country.[10] Article 5 of the 2018 declaration says that:

> Each country or jurisdiction should develop and implement legislation and regulations to govern the recovery of organs from deceased and living donors and the practice of transplantation, consistent with international standards.

This is an important article because it seeks to create global legal uniformity concerning organ donation. On the one hand, the Istanbul declaration imposes on the various countries responsibility for self-sufficiency in their organ economies, especially by developing a deceased organ economy. But, on the other hand, it expects countries to adopt a uniform standard established in ethical and medical forums of representatives of transplantation medicine.

But can perfect uniformity of ethical codes be expected in as culturally contested a technology such as organ transplantation? It appears that the Declaration of Istanbul is satisfied with a fight against the most extreme form of exploitation in the power relations that can arise between the giver and recipient – organ trafficking. But as argued above, power relations, exploitation, and coercion can also appear in more covert ways under the cover of everything remaining in the family. To be sure, the declaration also refers to protocols to screen living donations and emphasizes the informed consent that should be obtained for such donations, but even here, the protocols for screening living donations refer mainly to a specific Western culture, and their application as a universal protocol suitable to all societies and cultures remains problematic.

Furthermore, the declaration demands legislative steps such as criminalization of those involved in organ trafficking, cultivating donations from the deceased, adhering to international protocols and standards, and so on. But it does not manage to offer an ethical framework for donor–recipient relations in living donations. It emphasizes protecting the well-being of the donor and informed consent but does not refer at all to the fact that donor–recipient relations in living donations express a very wide spectrum of moral relations, care, obligations, and duties. Can there be a suitable ethical framework for those relations?

To a significant extent, the Declaration of Istanbul reproduces the dichotomy of altruism versus utilitarianism and donation versus commerce. It denounces the most extreme form of trafficking but does not find a solution to other situations of coercion and power relations which might lead to "donation."

The Declaration of Istanbul marks an apex in the global economy of transplantation medicine. It presents a detailed hegemonic position as to the moral and legal envelope of organ donation everywhere in the world. In that sense, it joins other international bodies that impose standardization, such as the IMF or the World Bank. The fight against organ trafficking through the Istanbul declaration is a process that can be viewed as a "supra-state" process. The expectation is, of course, for local legislation, and the analysis unit for the success of an organ economy is the state and its ability to provide sufficient organs to its residents, but the states' room for ethical maneuvering in the face of the Istanbul declaration is not particularly wide.

The local responses to the Istanbul declaration were not uniform. In the Philippines, for example, a 10% quota of organ donations for patients from outside the Philippines was canceled as a response to the call against organ tourism. But, a deeper look at the actual practice of donation after 2008 in the Philippines shows disparities between the official policy forbidding donation to strangers and the practice. But who is a stranger? In donations from the living, as we shall see in the following chapter, the range of relations between donor and recipient expands to the point that it is easy to forge relatedness. Such forgeries require a tight oversight system, which necessitates considerable resources. Thus, in the Philippines, a dual politics of transplantations was introduced: an official policy that follows the provisions of the Istanbul declaration and actual practices of organ exchanges whose legitimacy is questionable (De Castro 2013).

The Declaration of Istanbul operates as a global umbrella that seeks to dictate an ethical standardization of the global organ economy. But the global organ economy also operates "from the ground up," in the vacuums created by the globalization processes. If the Declaration of Istanbul indicates the decline of the sovereign power of the state versus international bodies, the organ trade networks indicate the decline in the sovereign power of the state versus the power of the new economy and the supremacy of the global capital flow.

Indeed, the market trade routes of the global organ economy are not unique and largely run parallel to the characteristics of globalization in the new economy: the dependency relations between the West and the rest of the world also characterize other economic areas, and the indirect connection between the hegemony of the consumerist world and the spread of chronic diseases such as diabetes and hypertension impacts worldwide public health trends. So does the movement of patients from prosperous countries to periphery countries for organ transplants for pay, the sale of organs by immigrants in the poor suburbs and backyards of the Western countries, and raids by organ traders among refugee groups and neglected areas of countries that crumbled as a result of civil war[11] – all of these phenomena are parallel to a certain extent to the ills of globalization and the new economy (Gonzalez, Garijo and Sanchez 2020).

Thus, in many senses, the global organ economy is part and parcel of the political contexts of the new economy. It is derived from the globalization processes and the global economic and political fluctuations since the 1990s. As argued above, the organ trade exists within the travel possibilities of the global world and the ever-worsening inequality and occurs in the vacuum created by the border-crossing movement of capital of the new economy. But, the organ trade is only one phenomenon out of a series of phenomena related to globalization, inequality, and medical technology. The most salient and widespread example of those phenomena is medical tourism: countries that offer advanced medicine in superlative conditions, or luxury medicine such as antiaging treatments, to wealthy foreigners (Cohen 2014). Medical tourism, one must add, often relies on public infrastructures funded by the citizens. In many cases, the citizens of that state cannot afford that elite medicine, and it violates the basic principle of solidarity and equal opportunity.

In light of the worsening of the organ shortage, especially in the 1990s, the phenomenon of organ trafficking increased. Organ trafficking travels the same underground channels as capital and various goods of the new economy. Second, the war on organ trafficking uses international organizations that seek to limit the political autonomy of the state in the name of Western moral principles. Therefore, both organ trafficking and the fight against it are only made possible as part of the global system that operates above and beneath the state.

The global organ economy operates in that way within the classical framework of the political economy: in a division between market and state with the correction of international bodies that govern the ethical code for organ donation, on the one hand, and with a market which, contrary to the hegemonic neoliberal spirit of the globalization processes, is a censured market. And yet, both the international dictates and the black market of organ trafficking are only two out of three sources for organ supply.

As we shall see in the following chapter, the family or the household economy indicates the biggest rift in the ethical order of organ transplantation because it is very hard to supervise its procurement mechanisms. At this stage and to end the discussion of the global organ economy, one can point to the main points.

A global look at the organ economy finds a hierarchy of core, semi-periphery, and periphery countries for organ medicine that differ from each other in their infrastructures and self-sufficiency capacity. Second, the most prominent trend in the organ economy is the rise of the living organ economy. Even in unmistakable core countries such as Spain or Italy, we see a significant rise in organ donations from the living. The meaning of this rise can be understood as a transition to private channels of organ searching. The political economy of transplantation organs indicates a rising trend of private channels for seeking organs. This rise has a critical significance for the entire ethical system of organ donation. In these private channels, it is difficult to supervise and accurately identify the motivation and the complex relationship between donor and recipient. The extreme case of turning to these private channels is organ trafficking, but the privatization process in donations from living donors begins much earlier, with the decision to seek a living donor.

Notes

1 See International Registry in organ donation and transplantation. www.irodat.org. The source of the data is the competent authority in each country.
2 https://nhsbtdbe.blob.core.windows.net/umbraco-assets-corp/1434/ldkt_2020_strategy.pdf.

3 https://nhsbtdbe.blob.core.windows.net/umbraco-assets-corp/7887/august-2017-living-
donor-kidney-transplantation-position-paper.pdf.
It is interesting too that in 2017, when the rate of donations per million was 15.6, the
target for 2020 was not changed and remained at 26.
4 World Health Organization. Regional Office for Europe, *European Observatory on
Health Systems and Policies*, (Bernal-Delgado, García-Armesto, Juan. et al. 2018).
5 https://www.americasquarterly.org/article/5-big-ideas-universal-health/.
6 https://www.ghsindex.org/country/brazil/.
7 https://www.scielo.br/pdf/ress/v29n1/en_2237-9622-ress-29-01-e2018512.pdf.
8 For each country, the raw data about the rate of donations from living and dead donors
per million people were taken from the website *www.irodat.org*.
A calculation of the relative rate of the deceased or living economy out of the total
organ economy in that country is made by an annual summary of the two sectors of
the organ economy and a calculation of their relative rates.
9 https://www.declarationofistanbul.org/images/documents/doi_2008_English.pdf.
10 Another innovation from 2018 is the principle of financial neutrality:

> Neither donors and their families lose nor gain financially as a result of donation.

This item was introduced with the principle of indemnifying donors for expenses resulting from the donation and financial loss such as loss of work days and so on.
11 Reuters (2017). Available online: https://www.reuters.com/article/us-mideast-crisis-
syria-trafficking/organ-trafficking-booming-in-lebanon-as-desperate-syrians-sell-
kidneys-eyes-bbc-idUSKBN17S1V8.

References

Alam, A. A. (2007). Public opinion on organ donation in Saudi Arabia. *Saudi Journal of
Kidney Diseases and Transplantation*, 18(1), 54.
Al Attar, B. (2020). Renal replacement therapy in the Kingdom of Saudi Arabia. *Saudi
Journal of Kidney Diseases and Transplantation*, 31(6), 1458.
Al-Attar, B. (2020a). Deceased donation after brain death (DBD). *Saudi Journal of Kidney
Diseases and Transplantation*, 31(5), 1163.
Albar, M. 2012. Organ transplantation: A Sunni Islamic perspective. *Saudi Journal of
Kidney Diseases and Transplantions*, 23(4):817–822.
Alghanim, S. A. (2010). Knowledge and attitudes toward organ donation: A community-
based study comparing rural and urban populations. *Saudi Journal of Kidney Diseases
and Transplantation*, 21(1), 23.
Almalki, M. Fitzgerald G., & Clark, M. (2011). Healthcare system in Saudi Arabia: A
review. *Eastern Mediterranean Health Journal*, 17(10), 784–793.
Arshad, A., Anderson, B., & Sharif, A. (2019). Comparison of organ donation and
transplantation rates between opt-out and opt-in systems. *Kidney International*, 95(6),
1453–1460.
Bernal-Delgado, Enrique, García-Armesto, Sandra, Oliva, Juan, et al. (2018). *Spain: Health
System Review*. World Health Organization. Regional Office for Europe. https://apps.
who.int/iris/handle/10665/330195
Björnberg, U., & Latta, M. (2007). The roles of the family and the welfare state: The relationship between public and private financial support in Sweden. *Current Sociology*,
55(3), 415–445.
Budiani, D. (2007). Facilitating organ transplants in Egypt: An analysis of doctors' discourse. *Body & Society*, 13(3), 125–149.

Boutayeb, A. (2010). The burden of communicable and non-communicable diseases in developing countries. *Handbook of Disease Burdens and Quality of Life Measures*, 531.

Cohen, I. G. (2014). *Patients with Passports: Medical Tourism, Law, and Ethics*, Oxford: Oxford University Press.

Cylus, J., Richardson, E., Findley, L., Longley, M., O'Neill, C., & Steel, D. (2015). United Kingdom: Health system review. *Health Systems in Transition*, 17(5), 1–26.

De Castro, L. D. (2013). The declaration of Istanbul in the Philippines: Success with foreigners but a continuing challenge for local transplant tourism. *Medicine, Health Care and Philosophy*, 16(4), 929–932.

Ghods, A. J. (2015). Current status of organ transplant in Islamic countries. *Experimental Clinical Transplant*, 13(1), 13–7.

Gómez, E. J., Jungmann, S., & Lima, A. S. (2018). Resource allocations and disparities in the Brazilian health care system: insights from organ transplantation services. *BMC Health Services Research*, 18(1), 1–7.

Gonzalez, J., Garijo, I., & Sanchez, A. (2020). Organ trafficking and migration: A bibliometric analysis of an untold story. *International Journal of Environmental Research and Public Health*, 17(9), 3204.

Grootegoed, E., & Van Dijk, D. (2012). The return of the family? Welfare state retrenchment and client autonomy in long-term care. *Journal of Social policy*, 41(4), 677–694.

Hamdy, S. (2012). *Our Bodies Belong to God: Organ Transplants, Islam, and the Struggle for Human Dignity in Egypt*, California: University of California Press.

Mobaraki, A. E. H., & Soderfeldt, B. (2010). Gender inequity in Saudi Arabia and its role in public health. *EMHJ – Eastern Mediterranean Health Journal*, 16(1), 113–118.

Moosa, M. R. (2019). The state of kidney transplantation in South Africa. *South African Medical Journal*, 109(4), 235–240.

Muller, E., White, S., & Delmonico, F. (2014). Regional perspective: developing organ transplantation in sub-Saharan Africa. *Transplantation*, 97(10), 975–976.

Naicker, S. (2009). End-stage renal disease in sub-Saharan Africa. *Ethnicity & Disease*, 19(1), 13.

Oakland, W. H. (1987). "Theory of public goods", in Auerbach, A.J. & Feldstein, M (eds) *Handbook of Public Economics* (Vol. 2). Elsevier. pp. 485–535.

Papadopoulos, T., & Roumpakis, A. (2019). Family as a socio-economic actor in the political economy of welfare. *Social Policy Review*, 31, 243–266.

Powell, M. (ed) (2007). *Understanding the Mixed Economy of Welfare*, Bristol: Bristol University Press.

Sanal, A. (2004). "Robin Hood" of techno-Turkey or organ trafficking in the state of ethical beings. *Culture, Medicine and Psychiatry*, 28(3), 281–309.

Scheper-Hughes, N. (2005). Organs without borders. *Foreign Policy*, 146, 26.

Shaheen, F. A., Al-Attar, B., Follero, P. M., & Kamal, M. (2017). Critical pathways of deceased organ donation in Saudi Arabia: A two decades in comparison: 1997–2006 vs. 2007–2016. *Transplantation*, 101, S122.

Valentin, M., Mahillo, B. B., Martinez, I. I. et al. (2018). Living kidney donation in Spain, a global strategy to increase this modality of transplantation. *Transplantation*, 102, S133.

Wallerstein, I. (2004). *World-Systems Analysis*, Durham: Duke University Press.

5 The New Ethics of Organ Donation

The rise of the living organ economy represents a significant change in the ethical basis of transplantation medicine and organ donation. At this stage, I wish to add another layer to the definition of privatization, as conceptualized in this book. It is not only the process by which individuals in need embark on a personal quest for a life-saving organ but also the ethical consequences of that process. An organ that arrives for transplantation through the deceased donor economy route is perceived as a social good, belongs to the public, and as such is procured and distributed by the ethical criteria of equity. But when an organ arrives for transplantation through the living organ economy, it is perceived at best as a personal gift, something that is privately obtained. The organ itself is a product of private relations, and as such, it is charged with different moral meanings and obligations. In other words, privatization is not just about the political economy of organ supply but also about the moral economy of organs sourced from the living or from the dead. There are different ethics that emerge from the sources of the organs. This chapter will draw the outline of that new ethics and emphasize the differences between it and the institutionalized ethics of the formal, public, and deceased organ economy. The rise of the living organ economy entails nothing less than a revolution in the ethics of transplantation medicine. It turns the search for a transplantation organ into a "do-it-yourself" project and leads to the privatization and individualization of the ability to provide organs (Healy and Krawiec 2019 for a similar argument). One of the sociological consequences of that revolution, as we shall see in this chapter, is deepening inequalities – not only class-based – but inequality of social capital: who can marshal enough connections to procure an organ donor, or, alternatively, money to purchase an organ? In other words, my main argument in this chapter is that while the institutionalized ethics of organ donation was based on the division between altruism and trafficking, and the inequality it had in mind was the class inequality of buyers versus sellers, the living organ economy is subject to inequality of social capital, the creation of social networks, strength of community ties, and different kinds of social solidarity.

DOI: 10.4324/9781003288886-8

Between altruism, solidary, and utilitarianism

As we saw in Chapter 1, "altruism" and "gift of life" are foundational concepts in the organ donation discourse. These concepts are in contrast with the materialism of the modern age, with the social climate whose prevailing assumption is of the possessive individual and the insatiable consumer. The moral code of transplantation ethics – based on the concepts of altruism and sacrifice – is undoubtedly in oppositional disposition with contemporary materialist zeitgeist. The privatization of organ supply, which marks an increase in private and personal organ procurements from living individuals, sets transplant ethics on a more individualistic basis: it is not organ donated to a pool to be distributed according to public guidelines of allocation, but rather a direct gift between two private persons. Therefore, the rise in living organ economy indicates not only the increase in the relative share of the private domain in the political economy of transplantation organs but also the redefinition of the concepts of altruism and the gift of life. As we shall see below, these new definitions of altruism do not meet the strict requirements of altruism as conceptualized in the deceased organ economy. They emerge out of the personal relationship between living donors and their recipients. They are not moral categories imposed by officials as a rigid ethics set of norms, but rather the outcome of social structures and interpersonal interactions. In that sense, the privatization in organ supply is also the privatization of transplant ethics. To understand the magnitude of this revolution, the following pages are dedicated to the historical sources of the formal ethical discourse of transplantation medicine.

As far back as the 1960s and 1970s, in the numerous discussions about the ability of the public authorities to supply organs for transplantation, the main moral axes of the organ economy were delineated. As seen above, the possibility of paying for organs was rejected out of hand, even though the issue of organ markets as a solution to the organ shortage was never taken off the table. The organ shortage was at that time lurking on the horizon. It can be stated that the shortage not only created the traffic of organs for transplantation, but also the moral axes delineated their travel routes and the volume of the flow through them. The moral categories that were found suitable to serve as motivation for organ donation were altruism and solidarity. But what is altruism, and how did it become a basic category in the economy of body parts, in general, and organ donation in particular? What is the nature of solidarity?

As for altruism, I will start with the bottom line. Altruism became a central ethical category in the political economy of organs for transplantation for two reasons: first, transplantation medicine required the creation of a moral instrument that would justify both the instrumentalization of human organs and their treatment as objects separate from the body and the harm to one person to cure another person. The use of body parts – organs, tissues, cells – as health resources for distribution seems like an extreme case of reification of the human body and violation of human dignity, and altruism sought to solve that problem: the act of sacrifice served as a sufficient justification, in a possibly surprising way, for the digression from the Kantian principles of liberal bioethics. Second, the transformation of the concept of altruism into an ethical category redirected the discussion from the question of the violation of the body to the question of autonomy: the ethical questions involved in self-harm or reification of the body are resolved by the concept of personal choice (in the previous chapters, we saw the shortcomings of this philosophy concerning the donation of organs after death and the dead donor rule).

The altruistic principle serves as a rehabilitator, a purifying mechanism – it allows organ donation to be consistent with the principles of bioethics. The ethical dilemma involved in harming the living body of a healthy person or using the body of a deceased person to donate organs is, therefore, laid at the feet of a private individual – and not at the feet of the physician, who is bound by the medical ethical code. The assumption is that there is, indeed, autonomy, namely, that the donation is made out of personal choice, without material considerations, without coercion or exploitation, and out of the full understanding of the ethical complexity of the situation. Only such pure discretion can justify the violation of the rule "first do no harm" and the instrumentalization of the body. The fact that sacrificing an organ for the sake of another person is result of a decision that runs counter to the assumption of the rational agent as self-benefiting and is exactly what underlies defining this decision "altruism."

In his works, sociologist Kieran Healy argues that organ procurement agencies actually encourage altruism. He argues, in reference to American society, that organ donation not only expresses altruism but also generates it (Healy 2010, 2004, 2000). For Healy, altruism is conceptualized as a closed behavior pattern. He explains it with game theory-like calculations, or through institutional and social elements such as the organ procurement agencies and the bureaucratic system, which turned altruism into a clear behavioral category and a collective ethical concept. I wish to carry Healy's argument further and show that altruism has also become a framework for justifying and legitimizing the procurement of human organs for transplantation even more than a descriptive category.

Much has been written about the difference between altruism and self-interest or utilitarianism. In fact, these quarreling twins appear in a joint entry by Alasdair MacIntyre in the Encyclopedia of Philosophy (1967). "The problem (of altruism, H.B) was not fully put forth," writes MacIntyre, "until the 17th and 18th centuries." The context, of course, is the emergence of individualism as the base unit of political thought. MacIntyre points to Thomas Hobbes as the starting point of the discussion of the relationship between altruism and self-interest: the paradox, according to Hobbes, is that freedom is obtained only by sacrificing personal liberty. Therefore, changing the unit of analysis, or moving the unit of context from the individual to the collective, is a multidisciplinary solution of the paradox or the irony of altruism: what looks like altruism on the individual level turns out to be a completely utilitarian action, which even reflects self-interest, on the collective level. When individuals renounce their personal freedom – according to the Hobbesian argument – they gain advantages at the collective level in the form of sovereignty and security. Interestingly, Dawkins' theory on the selfish gene ascribes the same logic to the gene level (Dawkins 2017).

The term "altruism" was coined by sociologist August Comte (1895) at a late stage of his writing, in an attempt to present an alternative, quasi-religious model, for future society. Comte, who also coined the term "sociology" and is considered one of the founding fathers of the discipline, wished to establish a social science that would encompass all of the sciences and lead humanity into an advanced stage of collective moral life. Comte placed altruism in contrast to self-benefit and egoism, which characterized the material morality of the 19th-century capitalism, and especially in contrast with material life in bourgeois Paris in that century. He emphasized that society is more than a combination of egoistic atoms and argued that its progress demands renouncing possessiveness, pettiness, and individualism caught in materialistic bookkeeping – "for the sake of others." Altruism is, therefore, defined by contrast with self-interest and from the outset was presented as an ideal aspiration in the face of reality.

Altruism in its primary meaning is an absolute term. It does not have degrees, and a single drop of utilitarianism pollutes it beyond repair.[1] This characteristic is expressed by ascetic altruism, Simon Weil-style, which seeks to purify itself of any materialistic feature and rise from gravity to grace by negating personal needs (Weil 1997). Altruism was born, therefore, as a moral ideal in the context of a modern and secular society, an ideal that hails sacrifice and renunciation of personal gain for the sake of the other. Although it bears traces of Christian ethics, the main difference between altruism as an expression of a "modern religion" and Christianity is that altruism stands by itself and is not necessarily testament to faith or a component in a larger theological scheme. In that sense altruism is a modern concept: it accepts as a premise that the individual is the fundamental unit of society but wishes to replace the possessive individual with the moral individual. A similar attempt was proposed by Emmanuel Levinas, for instance, when he turned "the face of the other" into the addressee of the human experience (Peperzak and Lévinas 1993).

Is altruism a form of elitism? After all, if it became the norm, the rule, personal sacrifice would lose its uniqueness. In a society where giving charity in secret is the normal behavior, an anonymous donation would not elicit the same applause as it does in a community where such an action is exceptional. That is the paradox of altruism: when it becomes institutionalized, it becomes a behavior pattern and is no longer perceived as altruism, except by an outsider. Therefore, altruistic behavior must always be relative and always exceptional. Its proliferation, establishment, and integration in society neutralize it. This characteristic makes altruism an elitist behavior by definition. For a particular behavior to be considered altruistic, it has to be exceptional, and it has to arise from the free will of the individual and not from a social norm. One might even take the elitist definition of altruism so far as to completely eradicate its feasibility. That was, in fact, the conclusion of George Price, the famous altruism researcher, who was so crazed by the altruism riddle that he lost his mind (Harman 2011).

The life and death of George Price are to a large extent the ending point of Comte's ambitious project. Altruism as a social positivist project disappeared, and the term began to serve on the theoretical level, in the study of human behavior and in the field of social biology. Altruism made a comeback in the second half of the twentieth century, precisely in the area of public health. Its main ideologue this time was Richard Titmuss in his groundbreaking book *The Gift Relationship: From Human Blood to Social Policy* (Titmuss 1997). Titmuss, one of the architects of the British welfare policy, presents in his book different methods of collecting blood donations. He concludes that the best way socially and most effective way economically to collect blood donations is on the basis of personal volunteering. Titmuss proposed a paradigmatic shift from a utilitarian to a voluntary philosophy, thereby founding the space in which the altruistic code would take root as a moral regime for the procurement of body organs and cells. He adopted the call to encourage altruism from sociologist Pitirim Sorokin, one of the leading researchers of altruism, who claimed that giving is contagious and, therefore, society must provide opportunities for altruistic behavior. Following Titmuss's conclusion, the blood donation policy in the United States was changed. Thus was created the first public health behavior model on the basis of a purely voluntary criterion and on the basis of the bioethical principles that were being developed in those years.

Two main points arise from Titmuss's theory: one is the use of the word "gift" as formulated by Marcel Mauss in the context of archaic societies. Mauss wrote that in archaic societies "to give something is to give part of yourself" (Mauss 2002:10). He mainly emphasizes the duty of mutuality, and the social glue created by the norms of receiving, giving, and the duty to give back in equal measure – all norms that belong to the economy of gifts. The second point is the emphasis on the autonomy of the individual and free choice. I argue that these two sources of inspiration – the anthropology of the gift and the concept of the autonomous individual from which his notion of a liberal welfare state developed – serve as the ideological background for the reemergence of the concept of altruism as the moral sphere for the supply of organs, tissues, and body cells for therapeutic purposes.

The association created by Titmuss between Marcel Mauss's research into the concept of the gift and the voluntary procurement of medical resources such as blood and organs became the paradigm for understanding the association between medicine, community, and donation. The gift, an ancient custom rooted in human society, is presented by Titmuss as a way to build an economy founded on social cohesion. For him, Mauss's theory of the gift is an ancient promise waiting to be fulfilled in the context of 20th advanced medical technologies that will foster social solidarity. Writes Titmuss:

> This book, centring on gift relationships, is an attempt at measurement in respect of one such institution (blood donations H.B.). It has also advanced three inter-related theses. First, that gift-exchange of a non quantifiable nature has some important functions in complex, large-scale societies that the writing of Levi-Strauss and other would suggest. Second, the application of scientific and technological developments in such societies, in further accelerating the spread of complexity, has increased rather than diminished the scientific

as well as the social need for gift relationships. Third, for these and many other reasons, modern societies now require more, rather than less, freedom of choice for the expression of altruism in the daily life of all social groups.

(Titmuss 1997:290–291)

Titmuss provides us – through Mauss, Levi Strauss, and others – with a horizon of hope for solidarity on a new order. For him, the blood donations themselves are not the heart of the matter, and nor for that matter are organ donations. Titmuss is looking for the path to achieve solidarity and social cohesion, and for him, altruism and voluntary giving are the means to that end.

The return to a premodern, pre-capitalist era, as inspiration for the appropriate economic system for blood and organ donations, is interesting. The context in which Titmuss writes is modern capitalist society, the bureaucratic state that translates cultural worldviews into practical tasks, whereas the anthropologists he relies on describe an archaic society with total social institutions. In a total social institution, the entire social and political logic, not only the social economy, is embodied in exchange. The act of exchange expresses the culture, the family, the religion, the politics, and the law – as far as these structures can be differentiated in archaic societies. Indeed, Titmuss wishes to update the terms of the social economy and adapt them to modern societies based on differentiation, individualism, and liberty, but at the same time, he creates an association between gift relations and archaic societies, as formulated by anthropological structuralism, and the modern concepts of choice, altruism, and autonomy – even though they are different conceptual systems, deriving from completely different historical and social contexts.

The quintessential expression of the gift economy as a means of creating social connection appears before us, in the era of alienated modernity, in the act of organ donation, the so-called "gift of life." The "gift of life" metaphor enables us to blunt the incongruence between the structural concept of the gift in archaic societies and the methodological liberalism of the modern West; within the gift discourse, organ donation becomes an expression of autonomy and free will. The free choice, therefore, is an individualization of Mauss's concept of the gift. In other words, the translation of Mauss into the modern world involved removing the overall social envelope extended in his discussion over archaic societies, in favor of a social economy based on personal will and free choice.

At this point, it is worth looking at the nature of solidarity and the difference between it and altruism. Solidarity is based on an action that creates a partnership, whereas altruism remains a mere action, sometimes unique, in favor of a stranger. Titmuss connected the two: altruism expands the boundaries of the group, strengthens its internal ties, and thereby leads to increasing solidarity. But the question is: does altruism lead to solidarity, or is it the other way around? Altruism is aimed at the stranger and thereby expresses a universal concept of a human being as a human being, and by doing so offers solidarity with all of humanity. But Emile Durkheim, the most fertile and important theoretician of solidarity, has already demonstrated that the action of the individual is influenced by a presumption of a certain social structure. He called it "pre-contractual solidarity." Durkheim wished to challenge the common notion that society is based on a social contract – whether à la Russo or à la Hobbs or Locke (Follert 2020, Durkheim 2014). He argues that a moral perception of the social structure is the "natural state" of human society. Therefore, a certain degree of solidarity may be a condition for the very possibility of interpersonal interaction.

The question of solidarity has recently drawn new research interest in the context of health policy. Barbara Prainsack and Alena Buyx published a report about the consequences of the concept of solidarity for contemporary bioethics in general, for health policy, and for the use of advanced medical technologies (Prainsack and Buyx 2017). The researchers offer a new concept of solidarity, based on the active participation of the individual in health enterprises for the common good. They view solidarity as a pragmatic concept: it is the result of specific actions or practices by individuals whose purpose is to reduce costs for others, such as consent to participate in research, donate blood, and so on. Thus, for instance, biobanks would be based on people's willingness to provide personal medical information on the assumption that building as big a biobank as possible would benefit the entire public. Thus, the solidarity the researchers offer is not necessarily based on values that precede action, such as empathy or generosity, but on personal benefit that arises from contribution to the collective. Angus Dawson and Marcel Verweij distinguish, in the context of health policy, between "rational solidarity" – namely, solidarity based on a calculation of benefit, in which the cooperation between individuals derives from the understanding that the good of the individual is derived from the good of the collective – and "constitutive solidarity," in which the sense of group belonging is the motivation for action (Dawson and Verweij 2012). In any case, both Prainsack and Buyx and Dawson and Verweij offer a new agenda that emphasizes the importance of the social relationship as the basis for action.

Gil Siegel and Richard Bonnie call for the substitution of the concept of altruism with the concept of solidarity, or what they call "a reciprocity-based social contract," including in the area of organ donation (Siegal and Bonnie 2006). They argue that the theory they offer is in the middle between theories that emphasize the utilitarian aspect of supplying organs – including the proposal to ease the rub of the shortage by creating a legal organ market – and theories that emphasize the collective element and seek to promote organ donation in the framework of presumed consent. Siegel and Bonnie think organ donation must be based on the presumption of mutual altruism: donation depends exclusively on the altruism of the other. This model resembles the pragmatic solidarity proposed by Prainsack and Buyx as far as the emphasis on action, and it resembles the constitutive solidarity proposed by Dawson and Verweij in terms of group affiliation, which leads to consent to donate. The resemblance to constitutive solidarity is the weak point of Siegel and Bonnie's model because the entire model is based on the assumption that consent to donate can be based on overall solidarity. It is hard to imagine such solidarity in the context of capitalist Western society, let alone in the context of the United States, which is the subject of their article. The concern is that solidarity will be restricted to the framework of the club of equals, namely, a homogenous social group in terms of resources and access.

The emphasis on practice, especially for Prainsack and Buyx, is relevant to our discussion because the action takes us from the realm of ethics to the realm of the politics of social relations. Solidarity is not a value that stands alone but is the result of social contexts and specific actions. Therefore, it involves both creating a social connection and creating social boundaries. Solidary means inclusion, but no less, exclusion.

Titmuss distinguishes between the economic person and the social person: one is guided by a utilitarian principle and the other is guided by the principles of altruism and solidarity. Consequently, he distinguishes between economic policy and social policy. He says that unlike economic policy, social policy is constantly concerned with the question "who is my stranger?" Therefore, it creates institutions and processes that encourage the sense of identity, participation, and belonging; prevent the sense of alienation; and enable the individual to express altruism (Titmuss 1997:174). Therefore, for Titmuss, solidarity is the act of creating a collective.

In conclusion, the differences between altruism and solidarity arise from different dispositions within the social sphere. The act of the altruist is not connected to the sense of solidarity and is not limited to the boundaries of their immediate affiliation group. The altruist goes beyond the normative action sometimes to the point of supererogation (going beyond the call of moral duty), such as the act of donating a kidney from a living person to a complete stranger. Indeed, the institutionalization of the altruistic action leads to the dissipation of the altruism and the rise of binding normative solidarity, but organ donation from the living is far from being institutionalized and, therefore, the concept of altruism is suitable in this case. But, it is not always a matter of pure altruism. The donation of an organ of a living person may be subject to various stipulations and takes place in the context of social institutions, political bodies, and familial and market logics of action. All of these, in Simon Weil's terms, impede the rise from gravity to grace.

I argue that the ethical foundations of organ donation as presented above are undermined by the transition to a living organ economy. In the deceased organ economy, the ethical framework of donation for the greater good is fixed. The social relationship between the donor (or donating family) and the recipient is brokered by the state, and the social roles of recipient and donor have a relatively narrow range. In the deceased donor economy, therefore, the donation is unique and anonymous, there is no history of social relations between the donor and the recipient before the donation, and often, there will be no clear future relationship between them either. Conversely, the living organ economy is wholly based on relatedness, and this concept has expanded to include an increasing range of social relationships, which, in turn, create different ethical obligations between donor and recipient, which are not always identical to the definitions of altruism and gift of life as developed on the basis of the deceased donor economy.

Is blood thicker than water? The ethics of relatedness

Ahead of writing this book, I went back to interviews I conducted with organ donors who donated kidneys to family members and tried to understand the family dynamics before and after the donation.[2] I interviewed 25 such relatives and included diverse family relations between donor and recipient so that they included donations by parents to their children, children to their parents, siblings, spouses, and even more distant relatives. For comparison, I also interviewed donors from outside the family circle, who donated to people who needed a transplant and with whom they had prior acquaintance. It was easy for me to gain their confidence as someone who also underwent the process of transplantation and they opened their hearts for me, telling me their inner secrets of the donation process and helping me portray a sketch of transplant relatedness. In her work on organ donations in Mexico, Megan Crowley-Matoka (2016) describes the metamorphosis of the organs themselves as they are charged with the meaning of relatedness:

> The first key stage in the social life of a potentially transplantable organ, the very possibility of donation thus profoundly changes the meaning and value of other people's bodies for patients, for medical staff, and for family members (now rendered "potential donors") themselves. And once hailed in this way as potential donors, there was no going back to the time before when one's kidneys were simply one's own in an unexamined and undifferentiated way.
>
> (Crowley-Matoka 2016:197)

This observation confirms both with the methodology suggested here to focus on the transplanted organs themselves as carrying shifting meanings and values and in the sociological category of the family as it stirs different forms of kinship and relatedness. As we shall see, there is a sort of a dialogue between the organs and the social standing of those who bear them, mostly in terms of gender relations and roles in the family that result in the making of new forms of relatedness and in what Crowley-Matoka (2016) calls "familial sacrifice." Mostly, I am interested here in the looping of these relatedness constellations to understand the new ethics that is emerging in living organ donations.

The family structure and its roles is a crucial component in the division of decision-making processes regarding the living donation. Thus, for instance, says D., a mother who donated a kidney to her daughter, who was born with kidney failure that worsened after her marriage, to the point of needing a transplant or dialysis:

ME: Who is in your decision-making system?

D.: It was me, my husband, my daughter [who needs the transplant], and her husband. Just the four of us.

ME: And did you tell your other children?

D.: We didn't tell anyone until the time of the operation. I told my eldest son two weeks before the surgery. Only two weeks before. I told my brothers only after I was a match, because I needed some support. I told them only after it worked out (that there was a match) (HB). But, thank God, it did work out. They gave me the green light and we decided. I said, I will not let her do dialysis.

ME: Was your daughter part of this process?

D.:   Of course.

ME: Did she say, I want you to donate to me?

D.:   She… she… she… I knew it had to be someone from the family and not someone from the outside, because they said you could do it, at the time you could do it (transplants) in the Philippines, and she said: Mom, I would rather if it were you or Dad. And I said: I don't know if I will be a match. But thank God, He heard her prayers and I was a match and I donated.

ME: And did her husband offer to be the donor?

D.:   Her husband did it (the compatibility test) secretly. Like, he went and checked his blood type alone, yes (chuckles). We didn't know. And then he came and said mine is A and she's B, so so much for that. Even though I wouldn't have let him donate, I wouldn't have agreed.

ME: Why not?

D.:   Because, listen, I don't know what the consequences of the surgery are. And what can happen in the future. And he has no commitments. Besides being her husband, he has no major commitments. They don't have children yet. So I don't want it. I don't know how she would have come out of all of this. Today, thank God, she's healthy, thriving, everything is fine, but I don't know how it would have been after the surgery. So I didn't want to take responsibility.

As we can see, the donation story is intertwined with the family's personal history and has to do with the normative expectations from each member of the family. The need for a kidney not only created a crisis but also emphasized the familial division of labor in which, according to the interview, the mother played a central role. The decision-making was navigated by the donating mother, and it was she who accompanied her daughter from the first stages of the diagnosis of the disease in her childhood. She learned that her son-in-law had done a blood test to find out if he was a match for donation but stated she would not have allowed him to donate. The possibility of turning to the Filipino organ market is mentioned, but not as a first choice. The mother emphasizes she would not have allowed her daughter to get dialysis. All of the considerations, including the decision to have a transplant, the possible ways to procure an organ, and the ruling out of candidates for donation – all of that was regulated within the family without the intervention of outside parties. All the Ministry of Health could do was to approve or disapprove the donation.

As I said, the ethical point of departure is that family members have a commitment to aid each other. It is also surmised that the familial donor acts out of personal autonomy and free choice (Abecasis, Adams, Adams et al. 2000). The family is perceived as a closed ethical category and the family relationships leading to the decision to donate are perceived as a personal matter. But actually, the family is really an open ethical category. In the case described above, no motive is evident beyond the mother's concern for her daughter's well-being and health. But as we know, the family contains many possibilities of relationships, often opposing and conflicting. This can be gleaned from the interviews I conducted as well as many studies, which question the assumption that donations within the family are the product of altruism. Donations within the family are often the result of a complicated knot of relationships and difficulties (Crombie and Franklin 2006, Yi 2003, Crouch and Elliott 1999, Hilton and Starzomski 1994). For the recipient, the main difficulty – as we saw in the interview above – is merely needing a favor from their relatives. The plea for help is often silent and the initiative for donation often comes from family members. Second, the concept of personal autonomy and free choice come from the civil society domain and it is doubtful they are suitable for the family relations domain. The very concept of "informed consent," which is so central to bioethics, in general, and organ donation, in particular, is alien to the intrafamilial relationship (Gordon 2012, Valapour 2008). The concept is taken from the political imagination of the public sphere. It seeks to regulate the relationship between citizen and state and give the government license to use its power and authority toward citizens within the frame of the law. But the willingness to donate an organ inside the family is informed by a normative system of expectations, and we do not know to what extent it arises from an autonomous decision and free choice. For example, parents are expected to save their child (Zeiler, Guntram and Lennerling 2010). Spouses are expected to live up to the oath of "in sickness and in health" (Zeiler 2009), and siblings are expected to express commitment and care.

The relationship that led to the willingness to donate is checked by the pre-donation clinics in order to rule out the possibility of organ trafficking, or of coercion, exploitation, or fraud – usually toward wives, daughters, or sisters. But the inquiries performed by the clinics check for extreme possibilities, whereas the intrafamilial dynamic is complex and nuanced and is not fully revealed to the committee in charge of approving the donation. An inquiry into the intrafamilial relations that led to the decision to donate will find brachiated relations between family members, but the translation of those relations into the ethical logic of organ donation will come up against a conceptual barrier: the donation within the family is far from altruism, in many cases lacks the element of free consent, and the concept of gift of life is an excessive burden on it. Therefore, when it comes to organ donation within the family, the question of consent needs to be formulated on a completely different level: the level of the symbolic exchange relations within the family. Actually, the questions regarding donation within the family are questions about the roles of relatedness: should the family be the addressee when the need for an organ donation arises? If so, what is the commitment of parents toward their children? Of children toward their parents? Who is expected to donate? The discussion of these questions is largely divorced from the concept of informed consent as it is worded in the official bioethical code (Simmons, Marine and Simmmons 1987). The transition to the informal sector of organ donation, therefore, involves upending the assumptions of the accepted ethical order, undermining it, and voiding it of any real meaning. Instead, it offers a temporary and informal ethical system, which characterizes long-term interpersonal relations.

The figure below presents the family dynamics of organ donation relations as reflected by donation patterns within the family in the United States from 1998 to 2020. As we can see, the relations are dynamic but we can still discern consistent patterns: throughout the entire period, children donate less to their parents than parents to their children, and donations outside of the nuclear family are relatively few. Actually, donations between spouses are more common than donations from relatives related to the patient by blood and genetics outside the nuclear family. This pattern indicates the strengthening of the concept of relatedness as a social marker and the importance of the emotional relationship in such donations.

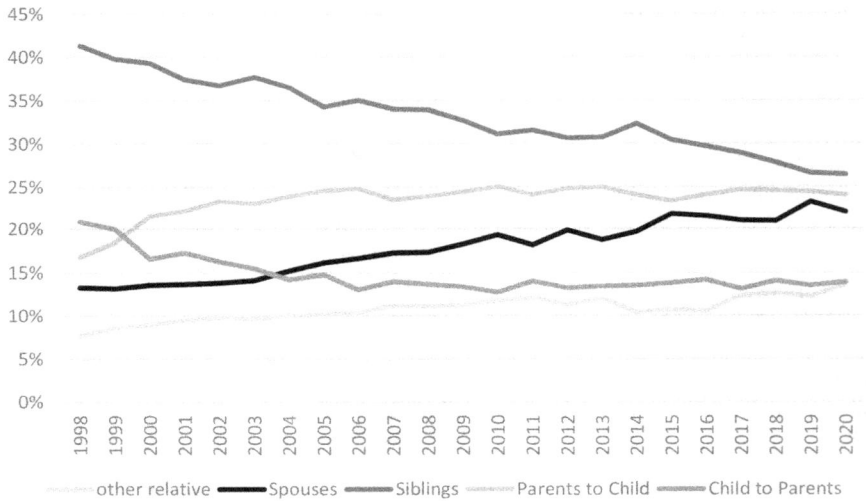

Figure 5.1 Donation patterns between relatives in the United States 1998–2020
Source: http://optn.transplant.hrsa.gov

Family relationships are not organized by the same logic as the public sphere. The concept of "altruism," namely, unconditional giving as an exceptional act in a utilitarian world, does not apply to them. Again, within the intrafamilial relationship, giving is the basic assumption and expectation, and not an exceptional act; self-sacrifice and acts contrary to immediate self-interest are considered natural. In the case of parents donating to their children, for instance, the donation is often conceptualized as "rebirth," thereby confirming the normative expectation system inside the family. Therefore, the definition of donation inside the family as altruism is at least not accurate and, furthermore, puts an emotional burden on the intrafamilial system as a result of the double message it embodies: on the one hand, the donation is conceived as an exceptional act of giving, and on the other hand, it is consistent with the normative system of expectations from family members (Crowley-Matoka 2016). Furthermore, since family relationships are ongoing relationships, which began long before the donation and are going to continue a long time thereafter, definition of the donation as an exceptional, impressive, and binding act of altruism might frame the familial relationship as a system of debt and thereby distort the relationship between giver and recipient and change the power balance in the family (Simmons, Marine and Simmons 1987).

The burden is always there. It could be a manifestation of the ultimate care, but the donation is always an act, which is acted upon what is conceived to be always the grateful patient. Framing this act as the "gift of life" creates an unavoidable tension within the family. The gift of life is a gift that cannot be returned. The anthropology of the gift teaches us that a gift that can be passed on and thereby create a chain of social solidarity. But inside the family, the gift is unique, direct, and intended for a specific patient with whom the donor has ups and downs, good times and bad times. In one of my interviews, without her husband present in a room, one donor, after 30 minutes of the interview, suddenly asserted: "do you know why I donated my kidney to him (her husband)? Because, he doesn't know, but I cheated on him. I couldn't live with myself and although he will never know, this is the reason why." I was totally surprised to hear her. Evidently, family roles yield different sorts of "gifts of life" and different kinds of debts. As mentioned, I, for instance, never thought that I need to act differently than my brothers to my parents. Sure, I try to treat them as a good son, but this has nothing to do with the kidneys they donated me. Only when I became a father myself, I understood their actions.

Relatedness begets different sorts of giving relations with their own specific ethics. In these conditions, unlike in donation between strangers, the gift does not create general social solidarity. An interview I held with G., who donated a kidney to her brother-in-law, illustrates why this conceptualization is problematic. I met G. in her small flat in a crumbling housing project in central Israel. Sitting in her living room, she told me her story, while she took care of her baby and her husband watched their other children:

> If I give you a glass of water you thank me. But something like this is a little bigger. The thank you feels small to me. Like for example she (her husband's sister, the wife of the recipient) told me after the surgery that she wanted very much to give me a thank you present. She wanted to design a custom made necklace or something like that, from a famous designer. I said to her, look at me, I have nothing on me, not even a wedding ring. I don't wear jewelry. Even if you spend 10,000 shekels on it I won't wear it. So don't bother, it would be a waste of money. I'd rather not. Also because I think I did it because I wanted to do it, I did it wholeheartedly. I don't want thank you gifts or anything. I would actually prefer, for example, if they were more interested in our daily lives, if they visited us more, if they shared with us more, if they invited us to dinner or things like that. I would feel better with that than if they bought me a blouse, or gave me 50 shekels or things like that.

After the interview, G. saw me at the door. At the doorstep, she asked me to come to her workplace the next day because "I wasn't comfortable telling the story at home." At our second meeting, she told me more about the relationship with her husband's family after the transplant:

> I give something important of myself so I also expect to receive something human back. To be acknowledged as part of the family. To be treated more humanly, for instance, when I ask them to take care of my children, because I have no family, I have no one here.

In this story as well, the donation is rooted in the family history, the power relations in the family, and the proximity and distance that are created in it. G. stresses the vacuity of material compensation for an action which she says she performed wholeheartedly. Material gifts cannot settle a debt created by a "gift of life." Yet, there is still an expectation for some reward: the real reward G. yearned for was her full admission into the family fold. Her shattered expectation of receiving that recognition casts an even harsher spotlight on the asymmetry of the act of donation. G.'s story is a good illustration of the fact that defining the donation as a gift that cannot be reciprocated impacts the power relations within the family long after the transplant (Crombie and Franklin 2006). Therefore, when it comes to donation between family members, the utopian concept of "gift of life" is devoid of meaning, and furthermore, puts a burden on family relations, creates tension in them, and can even distort them.

Figure 5.1 presents yet another interesting fact. The share of "other relatives" grew from 8% in 1998 to 14% in 2020. Who are those "other relatives?" Some of them are second-degree relatives such as uncles and aunts, but some can be "emotionally related donors." Mostly, the increase in the share of "other relatives" tells the success story of expanding the donor pool beyond the boundaries of genetic proximity. Originally, emotionally related donors are those who are not genetically related but have close emotional connections with the recipients, such as spouses. But with genetic proximity no longer an impasse, the potential for donors is unlimited, and as we saw above, emotionally related can indicate different histories of relations between donor and recipient. With even a more diversified pool of potential donors, the ethics of living organ donations gets much more complicated. The complexity of such donations is mostly evident in nondirected organ donations which is a living donation between strangers, as we shall see in the next chapter.

Ethics and gender: the gender gap in the organ economy

As we have seen, the ethical categories of the formal organ economy are too rigid and simplistic and fail to reflect the family dynamics that lead to donation. Moreover, these categories have a direct impact on the sociological structure of donations within the family. It is not for nothing that the donation stories cited above are the stories of women. The gender gap concerning organ donations inside the family is a clear expression of the power relations within the family (Biller-Andorno 2002, Kayler, Rasmussen, Dykstra et al. 2003). In other words, it expresses the association between the perception of women as agents of giving and sacrifice, and the perception of mothers, daughters, or sisters as candidates for donation. The concept of the family as a closed ethical category reproduces the gender labor division within the family, especially when it comes to caring for sick and elderly family members, a task that falls mainly on the shoulders of women. Presenting the donation as an act of charity, sacrifice, and a gift of life entrenches it in the traditional pattern, in which care, concern, and giving are perceived as the commitments of women.

Since the 1990s, the living organ economy has been comprised mainly of kidney donations by women inside the family. This figure crosses cultural, class, and social boundaries family (Kayler, Rasmussen, Dykstra et al. 2003, Biller-Andorno 2002). According to Eurotransplant, an international organization that coordinates organ donations between eight countries in Central and Western Europe (Belgium, the Netherlands, Austria, Germany, Slovenia, Croatia, Hungary, and Luxembourg), organ donations by parents to their children are the most common (more than half of all organ donations inside the family from 2011 to 2015), but mothers donated 1.6 times more than fathers during those years (Branger and Undine 2016). In the United States, women donated kidneys 1.45 times more than men,[3] mainly by virtue of their family position: mothers, daughters, and sisters. The main explanation for that was the perception of women as agents of giving and care. In her ethnography on living organ donation in Mexico, anthropologist Megan Crowley Matoka ascribes the gender gap to rooted cultural norms about gender roles, family, and suffering (Crowley-Matoka 2016). There is a lack of systematic data about semi-periphery and periphery areas, but we can assume that the more rigid and patriarchal the domestic gender labor division, the greater the expectation from women to donate organs.

Compared to the living organ economy, which is mainly a household economy, when it comes to organ donations from the deceased, the gender gap is the reverse: according to the Organ Procurement and Transplantation Network (OPTN), the number of donations from men is 1.5 higher than from women. Whereas in Europe, according to Eurotransplant, 55% of donations from the deceased come from men and 45% from women. The reason is a higher rate of cases of brain death among men. The reverse gender gap in the deceased organ economy requires a separate discussion. At any rate, this figure emphasizes all the more the gender gap in the living organ economy and indicates the depth of the systematization of the inequality between men and women surrounding organ donation.

The gender gap in the household organ economy is even more concerning considering its reverse on the receiving end. A study in the United States found that women have a lower chance of reaching dialysis treatments and receiving an organ transplant than men (Jindal, Ryan, Sajjad et al. 2005). According to the OPTN, from 1988 to August 2018, the number of transplants in men was 1.6 times higher than the number of transplants in women (456,652 vs. 282,785).

The researchers suggest that the gender gap in access to transplantation medicine arises among other reasons from a gender gap in the initial stages of diagnosis and treatment. Other studies found that there is a gender gap in access to medicine, in general, and suggested that one of the reasons for this gap is difference between men and women in perceptions of health and illness and their different relationships with medical institutions: women are more inclined to accept health statuses that men would have defined as illness, and men seek medical attention more than women (Glezerman 2016).

Therefore, the severity of the gender inequality in the distribution of transplantation organs reveals women's vulnerability both as candidates for donation and as candidates for transplantation. This twofold inequality sheds an even more glaring light on the incompatibility between the ethical logic of organ donations, based on the concepts of altruism and giving, and their political sociology. The combined action of those two factors might perpetuate the gender inequality of the organ economy. Given the internalization of the values of giving and sacrifice, on the one hand, and gender roles, on the other hand, what woman would disappoint the expectation from her to donate an organ? And on the other hand, who would upset the patriarchal order and wish her son, brother, or husband made the sacrifice for her? Of course, this is not to argue that organ donations by women in the family are not motivated by love and concern or that such feelings do not exist in men, but rather, to indicate the importance of the gender aspect of the organ economy, both on the giving and on the receiving ends.

The rise of an alternative ethical order

The incompatibility of the principles of Western liberal bioethics – and its concepts of consent, altruism, autonomy, and gift of life – with organ donation inside the family indicates a much wider fault line in the organ economy. It undermines the ethical order of the formal organ economy, mainly because of the direct donation system that characterizes organ donations inside the family. The ethical order of the formal organ economy arises from the principles of medical ethics. These principles take into account not only the good of the patient but also distributive justice, clear consent to donate, and mainly the desire to maintain the health of the donor. Conversely, the system of direct donation offers an alternative ethical order based on the utilitarian desire to save the patient. This ethical order focuses on the good of the patient and to that end relies on the gift of life metaphor and the altruistic code. The principles of discretion and self-preservation lose some of their importance in favor of giving and sacrifice. The alternative ethical order is clearly expressed by parents' organ donations to their children, donation that shows superlative commitment and expresses a normative expectation of sacrifice, and the utilitarianism that reaches its extreme in the genetic planning by which parents plan to give birth to another child in order to save that future child's sick brother or sister (Hashiloni-Dolev and Shkedi 2007). The only case where discretion overrides the consideration of the benefit of the recipient is donation from children to their parents. It is a relatively rare case in the household organ economy: according to Eurotransplant data, the rate of organ donations from children to their parents is less than 4% of all donations within the nuclear family. Parents will do anything to save their children; they will donate their organs and even have another baby for that purpose. But parents who need a transplant are not eager to see their children on the operating table, even if their children express the wish to donate for them.

Generally speaking, the alternative ethical order is the outcome of the development of personal initiative in light of the conditions of shortage. Personal initiative determines not only the identity of the donor but, to a large extent, also the time and place of performing the transplant, and coordination with the medical institution. When the donation is the result of a personal initiative, and is not attached to official waiting lists, the patient's environment has a much greater weight in making the decisions about the entire transplantation process. Therefore, a rise in the living organ economy means a rise in the weight of private initiative in the political economy of organs for transplantation. How can I get myself or my relative a life-saving organ for transplantation? That is the question that guides the living organ economy.

Following Zygmunt Bauman, I propose calling the development *privatization* or individualization of the organ economy. Bauman distinguishes between the citizen and the individual – the concept of citizenship is based on a concept of political liberty, whereas the concept of the individual is based on a concept of liberty without a defined goal except the realization of personal desires: "public space is not much more than a giant screen on which private worries are projected without ceasing to be private or acquiring new collective qualities in the course of magnification: public space is where public confession of private secrets and intimacies is made" (Bauman 2013:39–40). The private sphere, in consumerist societies – according to Bauman – is being individualized, privatized, becoming a projection of individuality.

In the late modern age, or the fluid modern age as Bauman calls it, "individualization is fate, not choice" (Bauman 2013:41). Therefore, the concept of citizenship gives way to individualization and privatization, not only of the market but also of politics, culture, and democracy. Bauman points to the disappointment from the state welfare mechanisms and the birth of a new individualism that creates, as a personal project, its own health, education, and even security services, services which in the past were provided by the state. Private regulation, argues Bauman, crumbles society into a collection of individuals who see reality through the prism of their personal benefit.

In Bauman's terms, it can be stated that given the organ shortage, the individualization of the organ economy is inevitable and has the capacity to undermine the ethical order of transplantation medicine. The extreme expression of that process is organ trafficking, but as we have seen, individualization is expressed by private initiative, in general – whether the initiative of the patient or the initiative of the family in its search for a transplantation organ. However, one must qualify that and say that the family might prevent the radicalization of the privatization processes down to the individual level: family members are subject to mutual expectations and unwritten rules. Second, the family might make decisions that are contrary to the wishes of the patient, such as to turn to the organ market.

Alternative channels of organ procurement

Indeed, the living organ economy is comprised mainly of kidney donations inside the family. But, over the years, a new trend has emerged, of increasing reliance on alternative channels of organ procurement. These channels illustrate the emergence of an alternative ethical order in the organ economy. Figure 5.2 shows trends in the living organ economy in the United States between 1998 and 2020. The figure indicates that organ donation inside the family is still the dominant element of that economy, although its volume is steadily decreasing, even when you include donations between spouses and donations from outside of the nuclear family (second-degree relation): In 1998, its rate was 91% of all organ donations, whereas in 2020, it dropped to 52%, a relative decline of almost 50%.

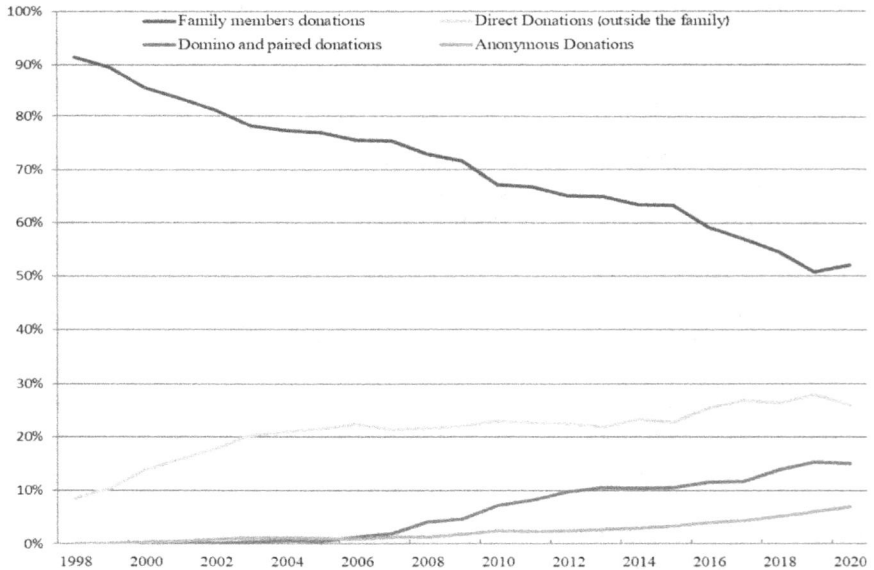

Figure 5.2 Trends in living organ donation patterns in the United States, 1998–2020
Source: http://optn.transplant.hrsa.gov

As the figure shows, one of the alternative channels for organ procurement is the crossover and domino method. Crossover or paired donations are organ donations between couples comprised of a donor and a patient. The donor in the first couple is compatible with the patient in the second couple, and the donor in the second couple is compatible with the patient in the first couple. Another novel method is the domino method, in which a donor begins a chain of donations.

Both of these methods are accelerating: in 2012, the rate of donations in these methods was already 10% of all organ donations from live donors in the United States, and by 2020, it had reached 15%.[4] Another channel is direct donation outside of the family. These are donations whose source is friends, acquaintances, and even strangers with some prior acquaintance with someone in need of a transplant. The significance of direct donation is expansion of the concept of relatedness to an additional circle of social relations similar to the concept of "emotionally related" discussed above. As the illustration shows, in 1998, the rate of these donations out of total living donations in the United States was only 8%, whereas by 2020, it reached 26%. These are donations mainly between acquaintances who do not share biological relatedness but have sufficient emotional attachment so that one is willing to donate a kidney to the other. Anonymous donation, where there is no emotional relation between the donor and the recipient, has also gained traction, and in 2020, 7% of all donations from living donors were from anonymous donors who were not acquainted with the recipient patient and, in fact, donated to a stranger. The increase in the rate of organ donations outside of the family circle is particularly interesting because it indicates the importance of connections and social capital in finding a donor. In that sense, the informal organ economy sector increasingly resembles other informal economies, where social networks and the ability to use and navigate them have significant weight.

An example of direct donation is the case of Y., 43 and the mother of two, who was born with three kidneys and donated one of her kidneys. The idea to donate occurred to her when she saw an advertisement by someone looking for a kidney. Following is a segment of a conversation I had with her a few years after her donation:

ME: Who did you meet, the patient?

Y.: Yes, the patient. He's responsible for all of the recreational activities in our village. I just wanted to ask what this was all about. He started telling me that he was sick. I didn't understand, I never knew anything about it, I wasn't interested.

ME: That was three years ago, right?

Y.: Yes. And then he said: I'm looking for someone to donate to me, I'm looking, I have to, and he's young, 55, and he says I'm willing to compensate them, and I'm willing to do this and that. You know, I went home, I went on the Internet, just out of curiosity, I started reading about what this is about. And those cards (donor cards), I didn't even know what that is, and I got cold feet, and I said like, as if I were going backwards, I didn't want to, I said I'm not going to touch my body, I don't want to, not going there."

"About a year later […] I was with my mother in a town in the south. My mother's family, a distant relative, we spent one weekend there. M., to whom I ultimately donated, came over, and said that she began dialysis and is looking for a kidney donation. It reminded me that story when I considered a donation, and I started asking all kinds of questions. And then she said she wants her life, she doesn't want to die, and she's looking for a donor, she asked everyone in the family. And nobody's blood type was compatible with hers".

ME: What blood type is she?

Y.: O and I'm also O negative.

ME: Which is very rare.

Y.: Right.

ME: Yes. It is.

Y.: And then I came home and said to Yossi, Yossi is my husband, I said poor thing, I feel so bad for her, what a shame, let's see, I want to donate to her.

ME: You didn't know you were compatible.

Y.: No. I didn't know.

ME: You only knew you had three kidneys.

Y.: Yes. I did know that, yes. And then he said to me, do whatever you want, I support you. Decide what you want. So I called her, I said let's meet.

Y. found out she was compatible and donated to M. Like G., whose story appeared above, Y. refused to accept the monetary compensation M. wanted to give her. Y. preferred M. over the first patient, among other reasons because of the timing: at the time she met him, she was not yet determined to donate and she needed more time, in which she resolved to do so. Furthermore, she sympathized with M., and a personal relationship developed between them that did not develop with the first patient. We must remember that contrary to the deceased organ economy, where anonymity is a ground rule, in the living organ economy donation to a stranger is perceived as strange and mysterious. It is inconsistent with the utilitarian concept of the household organ economy, and is suspected of ulterior motives, primarily a material motive. This is evident from Y.'s comments, when she told about her difficulty facing the committee in charge of approving donations:

Y.: I want to tell you, today I'm past that. If you're not emotionally strong you drop out in the middle. It requires a lot of emotional steel, from one committee to another, it's nerve-racking, and the pressure you're under, it's hard. And when they told me you need a committee, I said: what do I even need that for? Today I say yes, you do. Because anyone who's a little weak drops out, you can't stand it [...] I was strong so that she would get her life. So that's it, we got through the last committee and it was rehearsals every day.

ME: You did rehearsals with each other?

Y.: We talked. Every day.

ME: Role-playing?

Y.: Simulations. What they would say and what I would answer, so I wouldn't be stressed. So, the last committee was very stressful, and we passed.

ME: How did you do those simulations actually?

Y.: I played the patient and she played the donor, and then she asked me, why do you want to donate? How will you stand it emotionally? To see whether

I got stressed, if I could handle it, and then we did the exact opposite. And it's something that usually helps a lot because you calm down. I also went to see how she does dialysis. She did dialysis at the hospital. And I sat next to her and got an explanation from the nurses about the machine, I got into it.

Y. knew her recipient and came with her to the approving committees as a couple of a living donor and a potential recipient. Another alternative channel of living organ supply is the non-directed living donation, also known as anonymous donation, abovementioned. Unlike direct donation outside of the family, anonymous donation is to a complete stranger, although the boundary between the two kinds of donation is not always stark. The non directed donation pattern is developing on the edges of the organ economy. It is practiced far from the state procurement and harvesting mechanisms, which operate within the deceased organ economy, but it is also marginal in the living organ economy, which relies mainly on donations by family members or friends and acquaintances. However, there is an evident trend of increase in this donation pattern: as the figure presents, anonymous donations hardly existed at all in the US before 2006, but by 2017 had already reached 5% of living donations. As we shall see in the next chapter, this kind of donations have become very dominant in the Israeli organ economy in the second decade of the century and in fact Israel leads the list of non directed donations worldwide as of 2021.

Such donations tantalize the ethics of living donations from several angles. They feature the element of deceased organ economy where anonymity prevails the social relations between the donor and recipient, together with the fact that it is a living person who actually donates to a stranger. This combination yields a new form of donation ethics, where living donor has no relations with the recipient and their relatedness is only on the basis of some solidarity. Perhaps these donations are the clear manifestation of altruism with their immediate unconditional sacrifice, but it is specifically this direct form of altruism that render them contested and controversial.

While living anonymous donations are approved in the United States, Canada, Iran, Saudi Arabia, Israel, the United Kingdom, the Netherlands, Hong Kong, and Switzerland, they are prohibited in countries such as Spain, France, Italy, or Poland. This inconsistency reflects the ethical challenge they pose to the existent ethics of organ donations. Thus, for instance, Henderson et al. (2003) question the motives of such donors to be those of "lunatics or saints," emphasizing the radicality of such donations. In fact, Henderson et al. found in their study that living anonymous donors have a strong system of belief and faith in their act and narrate their act according to these spiritual narratives.

Hilhorst et al. (2005) warn against biases of discrimination and social injustice when implementing such donations. They note that "In societies where both race and religion have created deep conflicts, the fear of discrimination can be real indeed" and yet they add that "not all preferences regarding donation are based on dubious beliefs that exclude and humiliate. They can reflect a sincere and altruistic wish to help particular others." The ethical challenge for transplant centers is, therefore, twofold: to detect the thin line separating exclusionary motivations ("I do not wish that my kidney will be transplanted in a person from a specific origin/religion/ethnicity", etc.), from expressing a preference regarding the respected donor (I wish it would be a child/woman/first medical priority, etc.). The following challenge is then to decide whether to disqualify exclusionary donations or approve them and by that reduce the waiting time for a deceased donation to all patients. This, as will be explored in the next chapter, is the main ethical challenge of such donations in Israel.

Anonymous donation challenges both the utilitarian ethics of the informal sector and the ethics of the formal sector of the organ economy. In fact, it reflects the Titmuss logic fully: giving to a stranger by virtue of the ability to give and the very need. According to Titmuss, anonymous donation is the purest expression of a solidary society. The rise in the rate of anonymous donors is caused, on the one hand, by the increase in international and local oversight of organ trafficking and, on the other hand, the privatization of health issues and their transfer to the private sphere.

Another cause for the rise in the number of anonymous donations is the activity of the agencies that mediate between potential donors and those who need transplants. The Internet provides broader access to potential donors and patients in need of a transplant and facilitates the match between them. One example is the American organization matchingdonors.com. In January 2022, the organization's website listed more than 15,000 potential donors, including more than 4,000 potential donors for cross-matching or donation chains.[5] Matchingdonors. com is a nonprofit organization that declares on its homepage the prohibition on organ trafficking or any other compensation and adheres to the procedures of the altruistic dictate of organ donation. Those seeking organs pay $49 for one week of publicity and $595 for an unlimited time. Indeed, the working assumption of these organizations is that altruism does exist and that it has the power to establish a barter relationship that would supply the soaring demand for transplantation organs (Koplin 2015). But contrary to the anonymous donation in Titmuss's model, in which the welfare state is the only body that is able to provide the "opportunity for altruism", the anonymous donation of transplantation organs is the result of private initiatives, usually of patients who "market" their despair in the hope of finding a person who would agree to donate them an organ.

The tension between the altruism embodied in the anonymous donation and the altruistic code as defined by the formal organ economy is expressed by the existence of stipulations for donation. The activity of the anonymous donor is not limited to the personal initiative to donate an organ but is expressed also by selecting the patient in whose body it will be transplanted. It is a personal choice or system of stipulations, based on the donor's subjective social map. How will the altruistic donor select the patient they wish to save? By the extent of their need? Marital status? The patient's contribution to the community? Or perhaps by their religion or ethnicity? Those in need of a transplant of course wish to endear themselves to donors and attract attention to themselves. And in the absence of establishment mediation, the donor will act on their personal considerations and values. We will explore this new ethical venue of organ donations in the concluding chapter when discussing the nondirected donations trend in Israel.

Notes

1 In that sense, altruism follows the rule of the excluded middle; phenomena that have an either/or appearance.
2 The interviews were conducted in 2012 as part of research I did about motivation to donate organs among living donors (unpublished). The research was conducted with the transplantation department at Beilinson hospital and was approved by the hospital's ethics committee (permit 5878) and supported by the Israel National Institute for Health Policy Research (NIHP).
3 See data from US Department of Health, www.optn.transplant.hrsa.gov/view-data-reports.
4 These new forms of organ donations gain the attention of Nobel Prize laureate economist Alvin Roth, who planned the "New England Donor Service" which matches pairs of donors and recipients for crossover or even dominos chains of donations.
5 https://matchingdonors.com/life/.

References

Abecassis, M., Adams, M., Adams, P. et al. (2000). Consensus statement on the live organ donor. *JAMA*, 284, 2919–2926.

Bauman, Z. (2013). *Liquid Modernity*, Cambridge: Polity Press.

Biller-Andorno, N. (2002). Gender imbalance in living organ donation. *Medicine, Health Care and Philosophy*, 5(2), 199–203.

Branger P., & Undine, S. (eds). (2016). *Annual Report 2016*, Leiden: Eurotransplant.

Comte, A. 1851–4 (1895). *Système de Politique Positive ou Traité de Sociologie Instituant la Religion de L'humanité*, Paris: Larousse.

Crombie, A. K., and Franklin, P. M. (2006). Family issues implicit in living donation. *Mortality*, 11(2), 196–210.

Crouch, R. A., & Elliott, C. (1999). Moral agency and the family: The case of living related organ transplantation. *Cambridge Quarterly of Healthcare Ethics*, 8(3), 275–287.

Crowley-Matoka, M. (2016). *Domesticating Organ Transplants: Familial Sacrifice and National Aspirations in Mexico*, Durham, NC: Duke University Press.

Dawkins, R. (2017). *The Selfish Gene*, Oxford: Oxford University Press.

Dawson, A., & Verweij, M. (2012). Solidarity: A moral concept in need of clarification. *Public Health Ethics*, 5(1), 1–5.

Durkheim, E. (2014 [1893]). *The Division of Labor in Society*, New York: Simon and Schuster.

Follert, M. (2020). Contractual thought and Durkheim's theory of the social: A reappraisal. *Journal of Classical Sociology*, 20(3), 167–190.

Glezerman, M. (2016). *Gender Medicine: The Groundbreaking New Science of Gender-and Sex-Related Diagnosis and Treatment*, New York: Abrams Books.

Gordon, E. J. (2012). Informed consent for living donation: A review of key empirical studies, ethical challenges and future research. *American Journal of Transplantation*, 12(9), 2273–2280.

Harman, O. (2011). *The Price of Altruism: George Price and the Search for the Origins of Kindness*, New York: WW Norton & Company.

Hashiloni-Dolev, Y., & Shkedi, S. (2007). On new reproductive technologies and family ethics: Pre-implantation genetic diagnosis for sibling donor in Israel and Germany. *Social Science & Medicine*, 65(10), 2081–2092.Healy, K. (2010). *Last Best Gift*, Chicago: University of Chicago Press.

Healy, K. (2000). Embedded altruism: Blood collection regimes and the European Union's donor population. *American Journal of Sociology*, 105(6), 1633–1657.

Healy, K. (2004). Altruism as an organizational problem: The case of organ procurement. *American Sociological Review*, 69(3), 387–404.

Healy, K., & Krawiec, K. D. (2019). Organ entrepreneurs. *Duke Law School Public Law & Legal Theory Series*, 2017–2026.

Henderson, A. J., Landolt, M. A., McDonald, M. F., et al. (2003). The living anonymous kidney donor: Lunatic or Saint? *American journal of transplantation*, 3(2), 203–213.

Hilhorst, M. T., Kranenburg, L. W., Zuidema, W. et al. (2005). Altruistic living kidney donation challenges psychosocial research and policy: A response to previous articles. *Transplantation*, 79(11), 1470–1474.

Hilton, B. A., & Starzomski, R. C. (1994). Family decision making about living related kidney donation. *ANNA Journal*, 21(6), 346–354.

Jindal, R. M., Ryan, J. J., Sajjad, I. et al. (2005). Kidney transplantation and gender disparity, *American Journal of Nephrology*, 25(5), 474–483.

Kayler, L. K., Rasmussen, C. S., Dykstra, D. M. et al. (2003). Gender imbalance and outcomes in living donor renal transplantation in the United States. *American Journal of Transplantation*, 3(4), 452–458.

Koplin, J. J. (2015). From blood donation to kidney sales: The gift relationship and transplant commercialism. *Monash Bioethics Review*, 33(2), 102–122.

MacIntyre, A. (1967). "Egoism and altruism", in P. Edwards (ed). *The Encyclopedia of Philosophy* II, New York: McMillan. pp. 462–466.

Mauss, M. (2002) [1925]. *The Gift: The Form and Reason for Exchange in Archaic Societies*, London & New York: Routledge.

Peperzak, A. T., & Lévinas, E. (1993). *To the Other: An Introduction to the Philosophy of Emmanuel Levinas*, Indiana, IN: Purdue University Press.

Prainsack, B., & Buyx, A. (2017). *Solidarity in Biomedicine and Beyond*, Cambridge: Cambridge University Press.

Siegal, G., & Bonnie, R. J. (2006). Closing the organ gap: A reciprocity-based social contract approach. *The Journal of Law, Medicine & Ethics*, 34(2), 415–423.

Simmons, R. G., Marine, S. K., & Simmons, R. L. (1987). *Gift of Life: The Effect of Organ Transplantation on Individual, Family, and Societal Dynamics*, New Jersey: Transaction Publishers.

Titmuss, R. (1997) [1970]. *The Gift Relationship: From Human Blood to Social Policy*, New York: The New Press.

Valapour, M. (2008). The live organ donor's consent: Is it informed and voluntary? *Transplantation Reviews*, 22(3), 196–199.

Weil, S. (1997). *Gravity and Grace*, Nebraska: University of Nebraska Press.

Yi, M. (2003). Decision-Making process for living kidney donors. *Journal of Nursing Scholarship*, 35(1), 61–66.

Zeiler, K. (2009). Just love in live organ donation. *Medicine, Health Care and Philosophy*, 12(3), 323–331.

Zeiler, K., Guntram, L., & Lennerling, A. (2010). Moral tales of parental living kidney donation: A parenthood moral imperative and its relevance for decision making. *Medicine, Health Care and Philosophy*, 13(3), 225–236.

June 2020

Dear donor's family,

First, my deep condolences for your painful loss. There really are no words that can comfort and soften the grief and pain I am sure you are feeling. My heart goes out to you and even though grief will always be with you from now on, I hope you find a way to process it so that you can more or less go back to your normal lives.

We don't know each other, but my fate is tied with yours, and your decision to donate your loved one's organs changed my life. My name is Hagai and I am 47, married and the father of two children (ages 9 and 11). Your donation three weeks ago gave me a liver and a kidney that will enable me to live a healthy life, get off dialysis, and get back to my normal family life and work. For your donation and noble act I will be forever grateful to you.

This was actually my fourth transplant. Since childhood I had already been through three kidney transplants (the first and second from my parents and the third from an unrelated donor). I hope very much this is the last time I will have to have a transplant and that from now on I can live a full and normal life for many years. Before the transplant, my life revolved around my dialysis treatments, which may have kept me alive, but are tiring and exhausting and put the patient's life on hold.

Despite my medical condition, which I have had since infancy, I lead a normal life on all social levels: family, work, friends and so on. I am very familiar with life as an organ transplantee and it is immeasurably better than life on dialysis. Thanks to your donation I can finally get on with my life. There are no words that can describe my gratitude. Out of your grief and deep loss, you saved my life and the lives of other transplant candidates, and I think there can be no greater act of heroism.

I live with my wife and children in Tel Aviv. I have two brothers (I am the middle one). I work at a research institute on humanities and social sciences in Jerusalem. At this stage, three weeks after the transplant, I am still very weak and dealing with the consequences of the transplant (receiving high doses of medications that help the organs take hold). The doctors are happy with the results of the transplant and optimistic about the future, even though I am still in a challenging condition.

These should be happy days for me. I am indeed happy about the healthy life awaiting me, but I cannot get over the incomprehensible way that the tragedy of one family gives life to another person. As an organ transplantee, I am deeply cognizant of how our lives are always intertwined with the lives of others. This insight is always true.

DOI: 10.4324/9781003288886-9

We are not lone islands in the stream but always woven into the wishes, abilities, desires and fates of those around us. Organ donation emphasizes that principle: we don't even know each other, yet your donation was the most meaningful act in my life, which changed it beyond recognition. For your generosity, for your unconditional giving, for your ability - beyond the grief and loss - to think about anonymous others, I thank you deeply.

I don't know how this letter finds you. It is supposed to be a heartfelt expression of gratitude and to provide you with information about the heretofore anonymous person you saved and gave the gift of life. I don't know if you want to know more and how much openness you are interested in. Of course I will accept anything you decide. If you want to contact me, I am leaving my personal information below and you can use it or not as you wish.

I want to thank you again and to emphasize how noble and praiseworthy your donation is.

Sincerely,

Hagai Boas, July 21, 2020

The story of this letter, which followed my fourth transplant on June 27, 2020, is convoluted and entwined with personal dramas that are all grounded in the Israeli context of organ donation. My third transplant in July 2004 was very successful from the medical point of view but left me with the never-mending scar of participation – albeit reluctantly and to a large extent unavoidably – in the dark world of organ trafficking. Over the years, my relationship with the Israeli seller faded away and ended. He underwent upheavals in his personal life. One day, I called him to ask how he was. A woman answered his cell phone suspiciously. "Who are you?" I answered indirectly: "My name is Hagai, we were in Turkey together a few years ago, he knows who I am." "In Turkey?" she was surprised. "He never told me." I made sure it was not a wrong number and understood between the lines that the person I was talking to, apparently his partner, knew nothing about the story. Along with the tattoo he made in order to cover the scar of the surgery, all signs pointed to his wanting to leave this story in the shadows. I stopped calling him. It is now more than 17 years since the selling of his kidney and I hope for him that he is living a healthy and good life. I don't know how to think about my moral obligations here. The relationship between us was a personification of the dark corners of capitalism and medicine, such massive forces that there was little I could do to confront them then and nothing I can do now.

Medically, signs of chronic rejection started to appear in 2015. That year, a new medication appeared for the treatment of hepatitis C, liver cirrhosis caused by a virus. I contracted it from a blood infusion I received as an infant during my hospitalization just after I was born. By 2015, my liver was scarred as a result of that cirrhosis. Luckily, the new medication stopped the liver's deterioration but put stress on my kidney. In 2016, I underwent a complex urological surgery which also loaded an extra stress on the kidney so that from around 2017 my nephrologist advised me to "consider another transplant." The end of the third transplanted kidney was already visible.

This brought back the question that had been with me for an entire lifetime. Where would my next kidney come from? This time, my younger brother was determined to donate a kidney to me. He was almost 40 at the time, married, and the father of two daughters, and, at that point in his life, felt willing and capable to offer me his kidney. The initiative came from him in a kind of code of silence. The moment of truth arrived in July 2019 when my kidney function deteriorated and the transplant question became actual.

My brother came forth and the transplant coordinator scheduled him a series of comprehensive physical tests to find out if he was competent for donation. The tests lasted a few weeks and the transplantation coordinator was careful to examine every shade of medical doubt to rule out the possibility that the donation would damage his health. Surely, the transplantation system had undergone standardization and improvement since my second transplant in 1999. For my third transplant, no donor was found and the shortage was so deep in the first decade of this century that many turned to organ trafficking. Others lost their lives. In 2008, a reform occurred in the transplantation world in Israel with the passing of the transplantation law that provided a criminal penalty of up to three years in prison for involvement in organ trafficking, and the brain-respiratory death law, that fixed in law the compromise reached between the rabbinical establishment and medical experts on the definition of brain death. The history of the legislation and its consequences are described in detail in the following chapter, but for me as well as many Israeli patients waiting for transplants, this legislative reform was no great news because the number of years of waiting in dialysis for a transplant was not shortened. The Israeli public still lags behind in response to organ donation. For kidney disease patients, the alternative of transplantation from a living donor is an opportunity to escape from the abyss of the organ shortage. For other patients, who are waiting for organs for transplantation that come only from donors after death, the situation remained more or less as it was before the reform.

I remember well the moment when I understood that my brother was not suitable to donate a kidney to me. As part of the preparations for the donation, a compatibility test is performed between the donor and the recipient. The test examines among other things the level of genetic relatedness between the two in order to assess the chances the organ will be accepted by the transplanted body. That morning, the transplant coordinator presented me with the test results. There is, indeed, genetic relatedness, but there is a difference on a number of important markers that make my brother less suitable for donation. That was a shock for me, and I suppose it was for my brother too. I took a close look at the test results: his genetic profile compared to my genetic profile. This is individuality, I thought to myself. Right before my eyes, illustrated in numbers and in the language of scientific representation, is the uniqueness of each one of us. The possibility that genetic relatedness opens or closes to transplantation is, sometimes, so arbitrary. Here is my genetic profile, which is responsible among other things for the mutation that led me to the unfortunate condition of a chronic kidney patient. The genetic profile that I made every effort to avoid passing on to my two children. That genetic profile – which in recent years became a consumer product

for ancestry and family tree games for the affluent public by commercial companies that offer genetic profiling for pay –disqualifies my brother from donating me
an organ. Now what?

Now, I would need to look for other options. The first on the list: crossover donation. My wife and I had brought up to the transplant coordinator, ahead of my
third transplant, the idea that a donor who was not a match for me would donate
a kidney to another patient, while the other patient's donor would donate to me.
At the time, we tried to avoid at all costs getting caught in the vortex of organ
trafficking and the idea of an exchange appealed to us. We even advertised the
offer at the transplantation clinic (it was before the days of the social networks).
We received no answer. Nor was the transplantation coordinator very enthusi-
astic about the idea. By 2019, the notion of "paired exchange organ donation"
had already become acceptable and normative in Israel and the world over. The
transplantation coordinator found a compatible couple for such an exchange: a
patient suitable for receiving a kidney from my brother managed to find a donor
suitable for me. Her donor was unrelated to her. In fact, he was a stranger willing
to donate his kidney to a needed patient.

This category of donors deserves a closer look. In 2013, I published a study with
the transplantation department at Rabin Medical Center about the impact of the
reform in the transplantation law on the sociodemographic profile of living donors. We checked the demographic data of the donors who underwent donations
at the department in the five years before and after the transplantation law, and
we discovered an interesting finding: before the enactment of the transplantation
law, living donors outside of the family, who are unrelated to the patients, came
from a low socioeconomic and educational background and were mainly young
single men without children. We assumed that these were sellers who slipped
through the oversight committees at the hospitals. After the reform, that same
category of unrelated donors changed its sociological profile: suddenly, these were
educated people with more than 15 years of education, heads of large families
with more than five children. Men were still the majority, and they still came
from a relatively low socioeconomic background. What we discovered was the beginning of a wave that changed the world of organ donations in Israel. Groups of
ultra-Orthodox Jews who volunteered to become living organ donors to patients
they had never met and didn't know. The dry statistics we presented indicated the
trend but lacked the means to show the full complexity of the social phenomenon
that was gaining momentum in the second decade of the century.

From 2009 to 2021, more than 1000 volunteers, the vast majority of them
Orthodox jews, donated kidneys to people then didn't know before. In the following chapter, I will show the complexity of the phenomenon in relation to parallel
developments in organ donation in Israel, but at this stage, I wish to point out
the way these donors filled a vacuum that had not been filled by donations from
the deceased or the unacceptable alternative of organ trafficking which became
illegal in 2008. The donors are recruited by a nonprofit organization called Gift
of Life, which operates mainly in the religious Jewish sector in Israel. It is a private organization approached by hundreds of kidney patients in the hope to find

themselves an unrelated donor. The organization has a number of rules. First, it asks patients to exhaust the possibilities of donation inside the family and only then to turn to the organization. Second, it allows donors to state a set of personal preferences as to the identity features of the recipient. This point is controversial and raises objections. Is it acceptable for a person to choose who they are willing to donate to according to collective identity features? In this context, the issue that comes up is the preference of many of the donors for the recipient to be Jewish.

I don't know if the donor who was selected for me also stipulated such a preference, but the existence of those donations exclusively within the Jewish collective was clear and known. It made me very uncomfortable. Like my feelings about buying a kidney in 2004, here too I felt my identity gave me an unfair advantage. Whereas in the organ trafficking it was my class identity, in this case, it was my religious identity that gave me an advantage over patients who do not share that same identity with me and are left behind. I consider myself to be an atheist and conduct a secular way of life. That my Jewish identity will suddenly surface as a privileged status was problematic for me. The ethical discussion about the validity of preferences focuses on the positions of the donor, the organizing body, and the state. But, there is no discussion at all about the ethical weight of the recipient of such a donation. Like in organ trafficking, the point of departure is that in the race for life you say thank you to anyone who is willing to save your life. But, I felt a kind of distress. Of course, I wanted the donation and to save my life. But should I wallow in my good luck? In the privilege, I enjoy and that I didn't do anything to receive? What's better: to pay for a kidney or receive a kidney because you are Jewish? Both of those options are equally unacceptable to me and they both share the same naïve perception of a world built out of a series of personal choices. And yet, I could not say no to either one.

But fate put me on a different path. In a pretransplantation imaging, an aneurysm was seen in the liver portal vein. An enlarged spleen was also observed that gave rise to a different order of risks. The surgeons announced they were not willing to operate in this condition. The only solution they proposed was the removal of the liver and spleen and a combined transplantation of kidney and liver. Such a transplant cannot come from a living donor but only from a post-mortem donation. What would happen to the planned exchange procedure? From my side, it certainly was canceled and the unrelated donor would not be giving me his kidney. But what about the patient who was compatible with my younger brother? The transplant coordinator offered to my brother to donate to her anyway. Now, the ethical burden moved to him. My brother refused. He intended to donate to me and only to me. In that respect, like organ donations inside the family, he never viewed his donation as an altruistic act. He wanted to help me and, who knew, may be in the future, there would be no choice and he would yet donate to me after all?

So actually, the entire saga of my kidney donation swirled in a dance of stipulations: my brother's stipulations to donate to me, the double stipulation of the exchange donation, the unrelated donor who may well have stipulated his donation on the recipient being a Jew. This series of stipulations drew the outlines of the sociology of living organ donations in 2020: donation that is not universal but depends on entanglement of ties to the social positioning of the recipient.

I thought a lot about this during my dialysis treatments. Without a kidney donation, my condition deteriorated to the point of needing dialysis, and in November 2019, a catheter was implanted in my chest for thrice-weekly dialysis treatments. My condition was not good. My heart was edematous from fluids and there were weeks of daily dialysis to reduce the fluids. I was also put on a strict fluid diet that forbade me to drink almost at all. High levels of potassium and sugar also restricted my food intake. In addition to these difficult living conditions, the coronavirus epidemic broke out in Israel in December 2019 and added another layer of difficulty to life waiting for a transplant.

Covid-19 was a new threat to organ transplantees who are immunosuppressed. In the first stage of the pandemic, with no vaccines and no medications in the foreseeable future, the directives were to reduce social contacts. Except for dialysis, I did not leave the house, and my visits to the hospital, which was full of Covid-19 patients, were terrifying. I was on the waiting list for a liver transplant. It is a separate waiting list with different calculation rules from the kidney transplant list. Every two or three weeks, I gave a blood sample to determine my place on the list. Along with medical conditions, Israel has a policy of prioritizing on the transplantation waiting list donor card holders or people who donated or whose family members donated organs. This policy too violates the universal principle of not stipulating medical treatment on social behavior. The principal reverberates the concept of social worth, which was a criterion for distributing entitlement to dialysis treatments at the beginning of transplantation medicine and is no longer accepted. The priority principle was applied first in Israel and is analyzed in detail in the next chapter. In reality, when I got extra points on the waiting list because of my parents' double donation to me, I felt again how hard it is to escape the politics of the transplantation waiting list. Every channel of organ donation has a logic of give-and-take, accounting and stipulations that are piled on each other and on the structure of Israeli society, with its social, class, and cultural conflicts.

I was waiting for an organ donation from a person who died a brain death. It is a terrible feeling. Your ears perk up when you hear news of a traffic accident and you go into hyper alert when you hear about cases of organ donation. You go about your business and know that there is someone out there who is living their daily life without knowing that their future holds a head injury, brain death, or terrible news for the family that will show nobility and donate their organs. How can you even grasp such a reality? No movie, screenplay, or book can encompass the magnitude of the personal drama and the intensity of the emotions of donations from postmortem donors. Your luck is the other's disaster. To paraphrase a famous saying by Jean-Paul Sartre, it is not the other who is hell, but the other's hell is your ticket to paradise. How can you even understand and process such a terrible equation?

In June 2020, I was called twice for transplantation. The first time the transplant was canceled because the last tests of the donated liver found a problem in it. I was sent home instead of going down to the operating room. Two weeks later, an 18-year-old boy lost control of his scooter and received a fatal head injury. After a few days in intensive care, he was declared brain-dead and the family was approached with a request to donate his organs. In a later conversation, the mother told me how hard the donation was for her. In brain death, the body maintains its heat as a result of the artificial circulation of the blood thanks to the respirator. The deceased's chest rises and falls due to the artificial respiration and the decision is whether to turn off the resuscitation machines and lower the curtain on that artificial performance of life. "I don't carry a donor card," she told me, "and I got a lot of phone calls from relatives asking me not to dare to agree to turn off the machines and donate. But I knew it was the right thing to do." The liver and kidney were transplanted in me, and another kidney was transplanted in a Palestinian girl from East Jerusalem. The heart and lungs were also transplanted. Altogether, the family's donation saved the lives of five patients.

Three weeks later, I wrote the letter appearing above and handed it to the National Transplant Center, which gave it to the family. For the first year, I was in touch with the deceased's uncle. It was only on the first anniversary of the transplant, which was approximately the anniversary of the boy's death, that the mother wanted to talk to me. She told me about her son, her only child, who died in the accident, and asked about the well-being of his organs. "They are functioning," I replied. "They help me live every day, every hour." She asked why I had gone through so many transplants and worried that perhaps her son's organs would also ultimately be rejected. I tried to reassure her. I told her my life story. "It's an optimistic story," I told her. "I live in a supporting and loving family, I work for my living and live a full life." "I know all that," she answered, "you wrote it all in the letter." She wished me a continuing healthy life. Two weeks later, I read in the local paper that the memorial they erected for their son had been vandalized. I debated whether to call and express my sympathy. What could I say? That I am a living memorial? One mustn't think that way. I am living my life thanks to the donation, but it is important to be careful not to be drawn into being a living headstone to those who are gone. It has been two months. Will I meet the family? Will it not be too emotionally stressful for them? For me? It is hard to know how to behave in such situations and I am still wondering what the right thing is to do. My misgivings as an organ transplantee toward my benefactors never stop. They change according to the circumstances, the identity of the donor, the relationship between me and them, but the very receiving of the "gift of life," a gift I can never return, for which I will be in eternal debt, leads me to unending misgivings about the nature of relations between people, about our interdependence, about the arbitrariness that leads to acts of grace that save lives.

6   Contested Bioethics
The History of Organ Transplantations in Israel

The Israeli case exemplifies the crisis in the organ economy, at the same time, as it suggests alternatives for sorting it out. Israeli organ economy suffers from a severe shortage in organs for transplantations, as many other countries around the world, and it lags behind other countries with similar levels of medical services in organ donation rates. At the same time, it introduces, as shall be unfolded in the following pages, unique, original, and to a certain extent, unconventional solutions to the shortage problem. At a more general level, Israeli bioethics is famous for its alternative set of codes and practices. Its examples of Israeli exceptional understanding of bioethics, especially in the application of advanced medical technologies (Boas, Davidovitch, Filc et al. 2018, Siegal 2005). Thus, for example, the even existence of clinics for "population genetics" (Raz 2009) is unheard of in other bioethical contexts, the generous funding of reproductive technologies is again hard to explain as well as the incidence of IVF treatments which is the highest worldwide (Birenbaum-Carmeli 2004). Other examples can include posthumous reproduction (Hashiloni-Dolev 2015), the liberal surrogacy acts (Teman 2019), and more Israeli examples of regulating advanced medical technologies in a distinct way.

The temptation to view the Israeli case of organ economy as another case of distinctiveness and explain it solely out of its exceptionalism is great. But such a view would miss the opportunity provided by the case here to gain more general insights as to the connection between the bioethical and the biopolitical in organ donations, in general. I argue that the Israeli case illustrates, precisely out of its exceptional contexts, the constitutional problems and contradictions in the ethical envelope of the organ economy, in general, mainly in what was termed in Chapter 4 as core and semi-peripheral organ economies. Transplantation medicine in Israel, I posit, is an echo chamber of the global crises in the political economy of organ transplantation at large. But instead of minimizing the crises and hiding them under the cover of the rules of Western bioethics, as other countries do, Israel exposes them to all, places them on the public agenda, and offers them unique solutions. The severe organ shortage, the fear of organ trafficking, the coercion and exploitation that might go with organ donation – all of those burning issues in the moral economy of transplantation organs everywhere, receive an enhanced expression precisely through the local prism. Thus, for instance, the conservatism of religious circles surrounding brain death, on the one hand, and the

DOI: 10.4324/9781003288886-10

altruism expressed by religious people who want to donate kidneys to strangers, on the other hand, are good illustrations of the problems arising from adhering to a strict altruistic code. Likewise, an examination of the birth of the new altruistic subject in the local context might indicate the nature of that subject: their altruism is subject to a series of stipulations that delineate community boundaries, and therefore, the solution it offers to the organ shortage problem is local. That solution, which is inconsistent with Western bioethics, can help understand the crisis in the official organ economy in many countries.

A blurring of the boundaries between politics and bioethics also characterizes other organ economies in the world. But, in Israel, the collapse of the distinction between the scientific, the ethical, and the political is bared for all to see. The clear politicization of the ethical issues in Israel is the result of the public exposure of their internal contradictions due to the severe organ shortage. Moreover, the Israeli case also lays bare the blurring of boundaries between the public sphere and the private sphere concerning the supply of organs for transplantation. The Israeli organ economy indicates the ascendance of family and community structures as alternative political economies. Indeed, because of these features, the Israeli case cannot offer an overall solution to the problem of organ shortage, certainly not in the bioethical framework accepted in the West, in the core countries, but it can indicate the impotency of the state to offer an overall solution to the organ shortage.

Transplantation medicine in Israel, 1968–2008

The birth of transplantation medicine in Israel occurred shortly after the birth of transplantation medicine in the world. The first kidney transplant in Israel was performed in 1964, and in December 1968, the first heart transplant was performed at Beilinson Hospital, by a team headed by surgeon Dr. Maurice Levy (the first heart transplant in the world was performed in South Africa in 1967). The transplant was shrouded in secrecy, but word of the complex and advanced procedure spread and drew great interest. Besides the well-being of the heart transplantee (he died two weeks later following kidney failure), the question arose of the identity of the person whose heart was taken. The hospital refused to provide details about it. Avraham Sadgat, 35, died on the day of the transplantation and his family suspected the heart had been taken from him. Due to the hospital's refusal to confirm or deny their suspicion, the family turned to the ministers of police, health, and religion, demanding to know whether the heart had been taken from their deceased dear one. A month later, after being threatened with a lawsuit, the hospital admitted that the transplanted heart was the heart of Avraham Sadgat (Levy 2008, Weiler-Pollack 2008). No further information was provided about Sadgat's medical condition when his heart was extracted and the moment of determining death.

The hospital did not break the law when it took Avraham Sadgat's heart for transplantation without ascertaining his wishes, without his explicit consent, and without his family's consent. The Anatomy and Pathology Law from 1953, which was in force at the time, allowed taking organs from a cadaver to save a life. The first version of the law does not mention the family of the deceased at all. The scandal that broke out following the case drew attention to the harvest of the organ in what looked like an arbitrary act and led to the first discussion of its kind in Israel – parallel to discussions that had begun at the time throughout the world – about transplantations, the definition of brain death, and the ethical issues it involved. The health minister defended the hospital and argued the following from the Knesset podium:

> There is no doubt that [...] the management of Beilinson Hospital followed the existing law, which allows the use of a body part or organ from the deceased to heal a person, even without receiving permission and consent from the family of the deceased. When it comes to saving a life by transplanting an organ, Jewish law has no problem with that. Anything that can be done to save a life, we are not only permitted, but also obligated to do
>
> (Weiler-Pollack 2008)

Whereas the justice minister argued that "even in the future physicians in Israel must not be required to receive consent from the family of the deceased before taking an organ from a cadaver, although they ought to do so for the sake of peace" (quoted ibid.). The chief rabbis, Yitzhak Nissim and Yehuda Unterman, addressed the issue and decided that a committee of physicians and rabbis should be established to discuss the matter.

The Sadgat affair was the result of the ethical obscurity that almost always surrounds medical technologies at their inception. This affair, and similar cases in the world, reverberated because of the absence of an ethical framework to regulate the extraction of organs for transplantation. The main question concerned the connection between definition of death and the possibility of transplantation. As we have seen, for an organ to be eligible for transplantation, the amount of time in which the blood flow to the organ ceases (ischemia) must be as brief as possible. But blood flow means life. And how, then, can vital organs, let alone hearts, be taken out of people whose hearts are still beating? As discussed in the previous chapters, the association between the definition of brain death and transplantation medicine became the main challenge for the bioethics of organ transplantation. To a large extent, the argument over the definition of brain death is the axis surrounding which the ethics of transplantation medicine emerged in the world. As aforesaid, the definition of brain death by the Harvard committee in 1968 allowed transplantation medicine to use "warm" organs (whose vitality was maintained by the continued blood flow into them) of people who were defined as dead.

Western bioethics sought to create an absolute barrier between the ethical issues related to the definition of brain death and the ethical issues related to organ transplantation. Ethicists and legislators proposed systems of discourse and practical ways to actually separate the two. Consequently, transplantation medicine was regulated in international legislation separately from the question of determining death. At the center of the regulation of transplantation medicine were the issues of consent to donate, negating material motives for donation, and prohibiting organ trafficking; whereas regulating brain death was meant primarily to plant in the public trust concerning the determination of the moment of death. Although the chronic shortage of donation organs was marked in 1968 as the main motive for determining brain death as the moment of death, the question of brain death was, nonetheless, completely separated from the problem of supplying organs for donation. The ethical firewall between the definition of brain death and the problem of organ shortage has heightened in the decades that have since passed. The separation between the two became increasingly formalized, through procedures, laws, and regulations, first and foremost of which was the dead donor rule, until the association between determining the moment of death and organ transplantation was presented as merely circumstantial. In order to implement the dead donor rule, it was necessary to anchor the determination that brain death is not a borderline condition between life and death, but rather absolute and unequivocal death scientifically and legally, even though the heart continues to beat.

But in Israel, the contention with the question of the relationship between the definition of brain death and transplantation medicine took another path. Unlike in other countries, in Israel, there was never an absolute separation between the two issues and they conflated into one bioethical question. In fact, as we shall see below, both issues were almost from the outset political, and there was not even a serious effort to hide that. Indeed, for the health minister and the justice minister who backed the hospital in the Sadgat affair, the question of taking an organ for transplantation was not a political question. But that line of policy, which is consistent with the bioethics that seeks to separate science, ethics, and politics, was quickly abandoned.

After the Sadgat affair, transplantation activity in Israel was almost completely stopped for a long time. However, it is hard to know whether the scandal surrounding the hospital's conduct is what led to stopping the activity, or whether it was the general scientific standstill in transplantation medicine after the great breakthrough of the 1960s. As we remember, in the 1970s, transplantation medicine still faced the obstacle of the almost instant rejection of the grafted organs by the host's body. During those same years, a heated argument raged in the world surrounding the definition of brain death, especially concerning the precise site in the brain the cessation of whose activity determines death (Halevy and Brody 1993). The development of immunosuppressant drugs in the early 1980s heralded a global revolution in transplantation medicine and that is when organ transplantations were renewed in Israel as well. The renewed transplantation activity reignited the debate over brain death and the appropriate ethical framework for extracting organs for transplantation.

From presumed consent to informed consent

In 1980, the Anatomy and Pathology Law was amended as part of the coalition agreement between the religious party Agudath Israel and Likud in the first Likud government. It is not clear whether this was influenced by the Sadgat affair that occurred 12 years earlier, but there is no doubt that the amendment had a direct impact on transplantation medicine in Israel. The new law required the hospital to inform the family of the deceased it was taking their organs for transplantation but did not require it to obtain their consent. In fact, the amendment is consistent with the model of presumed consent and even spells out how one can oppose donation and avoid it. The amendment of the Anatomy and Pathology Law placed Israel in the group of the more permissive countries as far as its policy of organ procurement. According to the amendment, the consent of the entire public is a presumption that is not in doubt, and there is no need for explicit consent.

Parallel to the law amendment, the Adi Association to encourage organ donation was founded. The organization was established in 1978 by the Ben Dror family after the death of their son Ehud from a kidney disease. Ehud Ben Dror waited two years for a kidney donation, and by the time the donation finally came through and he was transplanted, he was too weak and died of complications two months later. The family viewed encouraging organ donations as his legacy. The Adi Association became an extension of the Ministry of Health and the National Transplant Center. The Israeli donor card is to this day called an "Adi card," after the late Ehud Ben Dror.

The presumed consent model as reflected by the amendment of the Anatomy and Pathology Law, the establishment of the Adi Association, as well as the development of the first kidney transplantation unit in Israel, at Beilinson Hospital – all of the foregoing could have placed Israel at the spearhead of the deceased organ economy. But the development of the deceased organ economy in Israel was blocked by the dispute over brain death, which arose from the refusal of leading rabbis in the ultra-Orthodox community to recognize the definition of brain death (Boas 2009). According to the way these rabbis interpreted halacha, brain death is not defined as death because the body still has aerobic activity (heart–lung), even if it is caused artificially (Stark Offer 2015, Halperin 2007). The very dispute on of the right interpretation to the halacha undermined public trust in the definition of brain death.

In 1986, the Chief Rabbinate was asked to weigh in on the matter. In fact, it was the director general of the Ministry of Health at the time, Prof. Dan Michaeli, who approached the Chief Rabbinate. As he would later recall: "I did not intend to get entangled in committees on this matter. I actually brought a done deal to the health minister at the time, Mordechai Gur, and he did not even intervene. He welcomed it" (Traubman 2002). Michaeli, therefore, presented the universal definition of brain death to the health minister and assumed the Chief Rabbinate would have nothing left to do but to sanction the deal. But contrary to his expectations, the Chief Rabbinate was in no hurry to adopt the definition and emphasized its weaknesses. Section 4 of the Chief Rabbinate Council's decision said this:

> Based on the foundations of Gemara [...] death is determined in the halacha by the cessation of breathing. [...] Therefore it must be ensured that breathing has stopped entirely in a way that it will no longer resume. This can

be determined by proving the destruction of the entire brain, including the brainstem that operates autonomous breathing in humans

(Kremer 2001:113).

This is the wording upon which the definition of respiratory brain death was based in the law passed by the Knesset in 2008, more than 20 years after it was presented to the public by the Chief Rabbinate. To a large extent, the law adopted the conditions for the definition of brain death as formulated by the Chief Rabbinate, as well as the rabbinate's proposal in that resolution to draw up a medical protocol including a series of tests and a list of diagnostic tools, all of which were required to be employed in order to meet the definition of death. The proposal to prepare a medical protocol emphasizes the contrast between the approach of Orthodox Halacha and the approach of the Catholic Church. In 1957, the Pope announced he had no intention of intervening in the subtleties of the definition of brain death because the Catholic Church gives the medical establishment a wide berth in determining the moment of death. Conversely, the Chief Rabbinate, followed by the Knesset, does not view the definition of death as a question concerning only medical science but also an object of political examination and consideration.

The rabbinate's decision also included an item that stated that the definition of brain death would be valid only if the medical team included a physician conversant with the halachic interpretation of determining the moment of death. The medical establishment viewed this demand as blatant trespassing and politicization of medical practice and fiercely objected to it (Reches 1996). This objection prevented the official acceptance of the definition of brain death for some 20 years. It is noteworthy that this definition was also met with suspicion in other parts of the world, such as in Japan (Lock 2002) or Egypt (Hamdy 2006).

Therefore, in the 1980s, the table was already set for the great showdown over transplantation medicine in Israel. On the one hand, the creation of the Adi Association and issuing donor cards were in keeping with parallel efforts in other parts of the world to establish an institutional and normative infrastructure for organ donation after death. On the other hand, the Chief Rabbinate's statement from 1986 marked an escalation in the turf wars between the medical profession and the religious establishment over the definition of brain death. Whereas throughout the world efforts were made to isolate the question of brain death and formulate it as a purely scientific question, in Israel, this question became a clear political issue. This development would become the most salient characteristic of the political economy of organ transplantation in Israel. The dispute over the definition of brain death along with the model of consent for organ procurement made it impossible to separate the question of organ donation from the question of the definition of brain death: objection to that definition was perceived as a sign of objection to organ donation. Indeed, as transplantation medicine became established in Israel, practices were adopted whose purpose was to distinguish between the definition of death and the harvesting of organs for transplantation. So, for example, a complete separation was made between the intensive care staff that determines death, and the organ coordination staff; furthermore, in the 1990s, the Spanish model was adopted concerning the transplantation coordination system inside the hospital and between hospitals. But this created only the appearance of resemblance to the Western bioethical code. Despite those practices, the question that concerned the Health Ministry, the Knesset, and public discourse was the connection between the definition of brain death and the severe organ shortage.

Transplantation medicine gradually developed in the world, and experience in transplantation was being gained in Europe and North America. The immunosuppressant drugs improved, and post-operative care was very successful in extending the lives of the transplantees and improving their quality. In Israel, in the 1980s, additional transplantation centers were opened beside the transplantation center at Beilinson Hospital. Transplantation surgery, medical follow-up, and the medications were funded by medical insurance even before the National Health Insurance Law was passed in 1995. The insurance coverage and the high level of the doctors and post-transplantation care put an even greater emphasis on the organ shortage. From the mid-1980s, as transplantation medicine became routine medicine in Israel, the only thing that separated people in need of transplants from actual transplants was the need to find an organ. The dispute over brain death was perceived as the main cause for the scarcity of organ donations, and the opponents of brain death were perceived as responsible for the organ shortage.

In 1993, the Ministry of Health founded the National Transplant Center. The center grew out of the seed of the Adi Association, and its purpose was to encourage organ donations. At the time, many organizations were created in the world to procure organs for transplantation, efforts were made to raise awareness of the importance of organ donation, and transplantation coordinators were trained, and in that sense, Israel did not lag behind the Western countries. These actions were meant to support the advanced medical array for transplantations. The transplantation coordination organizations, for example, can connect within a short time, and over large geographic distances, an anonymous donor with a patient waiting for a transplant, in order to donate organs after death. Such organizations operate mainly in the core areas of the organ economy, in countries that have active deceased organ economies. Therefore, the creation of the National Transplant Center was supposed to help Israel to develop as a core area economy in the global organ economy. Unfortunately, that did not happen. Despite the vigorous activity of the National Transplant Center, the rate of organ donations in Israel was then and still is far from the rate in Western countries.

As aforesaid, the low rate of donations is often attributed to the dispute over brain death and the religion–state relationship in Israel. But as will be described below, the matter seems to be related to the behavior of Israeli society as a whole, and not only of some of its sectors. Indeed, there is a stated willingness to donate, and the number of holders of donor cards is rising steadily, but there is still a gap between the intention to donate and actual donation. During the 1980s, and contrary to the spirit of the Anatomy and Pathology Law (even after its amendment in 1980), a practice was established of asking the family of the deceased for consent to donate, as is common in other countries. Therefore, Adi cards are not legally binding and de facto donation requires consent of the family even if the deceased signed the card. The card serves mainly as evidence of the deceased's wishes, whose purpose is to encourage the family to give its consent to donate their organs. Therefore, even before the 2008 Transplantation Law, the model of action had already been changed from presumed consent to a softened version of informed consent, in which the family's consent to donate the organs of the deceased is required. A situation, where, on the one hand, there is a low number of donations and, on the other hand, there is a brachiated and sophisticated array of transplantation organizations and transplantation units, characterizes the semi-periphery regions of the organ economy.

Geopolitics and demography: Israel and the question of organ trafficking

To understand the organ economy in Israel, we must add its geopolitical position and the broader regional context. The Israeli case shows how the informal organ commerce networks are built as part of local circumstances, on the one hand, and conditions of globalization, on the other hand. The frank report by Prof. Michael Friedlander from the Hadassah Hospital Dialysis Unit, which was published in the leading medical journal Lancet in 2002, illustrates how the shortage problem and the proposed solutions to it are embedded in the local geopolitical context, and how the shadow economy complements the deficiencies of the formal organ economy.

His words offer a rare glimpse into how the shortage leads to the rise of organ trade networks and show that these networks are created along the lines of the local geography, demography, and politics. It is a first-person testimony, in direct and simple language, that wishes primarily to indicate that organ trafficking is the inevitable result of the shortage. Friedlander's testimony, regardless of its normative aspect, is important to understanding the history of the organ economy in Israel and the growth of organ trafficking in it:

> Because Jerusalem is in the center of the West Bank, the explanation for this influx of new patients is related to local geopolitics. Before the onset of the Intifada (Palestinian uprising) in 1987, 92 kidneys (59 cadaver, 33 related living donors) were transplanted to Arab patients in Jerusalem. Since 1988, we have received almost no referrals of patients from West Bank dialysis centers, and monthly serum samples needed to crossmatch patients for cadaver kidneys have not been sent to our center. Because these patients were fully covered by the Israeli military authorities for hospital admissions and for outpatient follow-up, patients who had already received transplants continued their care in our clinic. Some Arab patients trapped in chronic dialysis treatment without the option of a transplant in Jerusalem underwent kidney transplantation from unrelated paid living donors in India and, more recently, Iraq. In a brief report, we noted the success of the transplants done in India, but also that patients were not selected and prepared for the

transplant procedure, which cost about $15000 including travel. Baghdad became a closer and cheaper ($7,000) option after the Gulf War, and we have reported on the first 80 recipients of Iraqi kidney transplants who arrived at our center. Again, patients were not selected, and our colleagues in the West Bank have told us of many patients who travelled to Iraq against their advice within 1 or 2 weeks of starting chronic dialysis treatment. Most patients who went to Iraq had met their kidney donors, often in the street outside the hospital in a group of competing donors. All donors were young, able-bodied men aged 25–35 years who received about $500 for their kidney. Our local Israeli Arab patients, who comprise about 30% of our dialysis population in Jerusalem, soon began to ask how and why their unprepared West Bank cousins and friends were receiving kidney transplants, whereas they, after undergoing rigorous pre-transplant screening tests, were still waiting for a transplant from a cadaver; and in many cases had been waiting for years. Here began my conversion from fierce objection to kidney marketing to passive acquiescence in this trade. We could not prevent our patients travelling to Iraq. We gave patients who asked our advice all the information I have presented here, and warned them that we could not help them outside our national boundaries, but assured them that we would immediately assist them on their return. Around 30 of our Arab patients have taken this option and all except two have had excellent results.

(Friedlaender 2002:971–972)

Traveling to Arab countries in search of a kidney was the preferred option for Palestinians on either side of the Green Line (citizens of Israel as well as those living in the Occupied Territories). Friedlander reported that in 2000, 29 dialysis patients went to Iraq and 4 to Egypt. Transplants in those countries were cheap compared to other countries. In the late 1990s, the Palestinian Ministry of Health almost completely canceled its funding of visits to the Hadassah Hospital clinics. According to Friedlander, the Jewish dialysis patients at Hadassah noticed the mysterious disappearance of the Palestinian dialysis patients and their return as kidney transplantees, and they too sought a bypass route to the arduous wait for a kidney. He added that, in the 1980s, Israeli patients bought kidneys in Estonia, Bulgaria, Turkey, Georgia, Russia, and Romania. At that time, prices soared up to $200,000 per transplant, and patients had to take loans or launch private fundraising campaigns to cover the costs. Ministry of Defense employees and pensioners received funding for transplantation expenses from the ministry.

Friedlander's testimony points to the direct political circumstances that arise from the military rule over the Occupied Territories. It also indicates the Palestinian uprising, and the Palestinian Authority after it was established, as central factors in shaping the informal Palestinian organ economy. In this sense, the health status of Israelis inside the Green line cannot be separated from the health status of Palestinians on its other side, as is often done. This case is a good illustration of Filc's argument that the relationships and power relations between Israelis and

Palestinians inform the right to health and access to health resources in Israel and the Occupied Territories (Filc 2011).

In the 1990s, organ trafficking expanded very much in Israel as a reaction to the severe shortage created by the scarcity of organ donations. The absence of a clear law referring to the source of an organ transplanted abroad; the wide insurance coverage for transplantations abroad (among other reasons because they are cheaper than dialysis treatments); and the insurance coverage for medications and postoperative care by virtue of the National Health Insurance Law – all of these lead more and more Israeli patients to leave the country and come back with a kidney in their body that was purchased and transplanted abroad. Data provided by the Health Ministry representative at a conference on organ trafficking in 2013 at Tel Aviv University indicates that from 2002 to 2008 the number of Israelis who were transplanted abroad reached 781 (compared to 459 surgeries performed in Israel). Thus, transplantations abroad, suspected as organ trafficking, were the main path to obtain kidneys for transplantation in the first decade of the 21st century. At the same conference, representatives of the insurance companies reported that until 2008 (when the Transplantation Law was passed) they funded transplantations for Israelis in other countries including Latvia, Russia, Turkey, the United States, Kosovo, Azerbaijan, the Philippines, China, Sri Lanka, South Africa, and Egypt. They also reported that between 1995 and 1998 Turkey was the preferred destination for Israelis to buy kidneys: between 1999 and 2004, South Africa was the preferred destination; and between 2004 and 2008, Israelis traveled mainly to the Philippines and China. The representative of one of the major insurance companies in Israel reported that, between 1995 and 2000, they funded 170 transplantations abroad for Israelis, and from 2001 to 2008, they funded 597 such transplants. The price of a transplant in Turkey rose over the years from $40,000 to $220,000; in South Africa, the price was $110,000 for the entire period; in China, the price was between $60,000 and $70,000; and in the Philippines, it was between $80,000 and $110,000.

The extent of organ trafficking in Israel, especially in relation to the population, turned Israel into one of the main targets of criticism of the international transplantation organizations. The international pressure on Israel led to a tightening of the Ministry of Health regulations against organ trafficking. At the end of the 1990s, given the trend of the rise in the living organ economy in Israel and around the world, the Health Ministry published procedures that regulated transplantations from living donors in Israel. A few years later, in 2006, the ministry forbade funding organ transplantations abroad.

In 2003, a draft law was submitted to regulate organ transplantation in Israel. The law was discussed in dozens of sessions of the parliament's Labor, Welfare, and Health Committee. The committee tried to resolve the problem of organ shortage while, at the same time, fighting against organ trafficking according to the international norms and regulations. The dilemma was evident: fighting organ trafficking meant worsening the shortage, whereas leaving the permissive policy intact meant, besides the price of allowing organ trafficking, also international condemnation.

It was not just another question of the allocation of healthcare resources in conditions of scarcity, the shortage question emerged as a primarily moral question of taking the organs of a living person in order to heal another person. For the international community, the transplantation organizations and the World Health Organization, the solution of the dilemma was unequivocal: there is no moral justification for organ trafficking and it must be fought resolutely. According to the liberal rationale of Western bioethics, the question of the shortage and the question of organ trafficking are separate questions. The shortage question must be solved as part of the education efforts and persuasion to donate organs following the Titmuss model, whereas organ trafficking is a moral wrong that must be fought without compromise.

Indeed, as part of the same reasoning, the distinction is made between questions involving organ donation and questions surrounding brain death. Even though the connection between those issues was revealed in internal discussions, academic articles, and even in the position papers of bioethicists, the separation between them is the hallmark of Western bioethical policy. In Israel, on the other hand, an opposite policy was pursued: instead of creating a barrier between the issues, they were thrown together into the political cauldron. However, as international pressure increased, it emerged that the permissive policy toward organ trafficking must stop (Efrat 2013). The solution was to solve the problem of the definition of brain death, in order to increase the number of organ donations from the deceased, so that the Israeli organ economy could become self-sufficient. Such a change in the model of the deceased organ economy could be made only by wrapping the issues of organ donation and brain death definition together in a joint legislation package.

Science, ethics, and politics: the package deal in the organ economy

The origin of the Organ Transplant Law and Brain-Respiratory Death Law, like many other laws, is in a personal story. Former Knesset member Otniel Schneller recalls that the idea for the law entered his mind following a conversation with his neighbor who needed a liver transplant and described to him the problem of the donation shortage. Schneller, a member of the Kadima movement who identifies himself as a Religious Zionist, wished to solve the problem by connecting the brain death issue with the problem of organ shortage. He made the association demonstratively, just like the Harvard committee for the definition of brain death in 1968. The utilitarian rationale for doing so was presented without embellishment, free of the constraints of liberal bioethics, which as aforesaid makes an effort to separate the two issues. Furthermore, that rationale is presented as the main reason for the act of legislation. The association between the transplantation law and the definition of brain death was meant to resolve the dilemma accompanying the discussions on the transplantation law for many years. Again, the purpose was to reach an agreed definition of brain death that would be accepted by the rabbis, and thereby to increase awareness of the importance of organ donation and increase the number of donations from the deceased. The Brain-Respiratory Death Law and the Organ Transplantation Law were passed together on the same day in March 2008. The proximity of the legislation and identity of those involved left no doubt as to the connection between them.

The Organ Transplantation Law emphasized Israel's commitment to fight organ trafficking. It set a criminal penalty of up to three years in prison for brokers of organ trafficking and the medical staff involved. The law also forbade insurance companies and health funds from funding transplantations abroad, which were suspected to originate from organ trafficking. Likewise, it established the status of the National Transplant Center and the status of the steering committee of the center as an advisory body to the health minister on transplantation policy in Israel (Green 2015). The Israeli Transplantation Law resembles in its format and goals parallel legislation in the world: it makes no reference to the question of determining death – although, again, its packaging with the Brain-Respiratory Death Law indicates the connection between them – and it emphasizes the prohibition on organ trafficking and the reliance on the prevailing consent approach (Efrat 2013a).

The Brain-Respiratory Death Law relied on a tradition of intermediate arrangements and arranged existing regulations, director-general provisions, and compromises. The novelty was mainly in the specification of the required procedures to determine brain death. The consent to determine death by the cessation of brainstem activity, which is responsible for breathing, reflects a compromise that had been reached back in the 1980s between the medical establishment and the Chief Rabbinate. In fact, the law is the product of years of negotiation between the medical and rabbinical establishments, brokered by the political system.

Furthermore, it is the product of negotiation within the rabbinical world as well – between the mainstream of orthodoxy (represented by the Chief Rabbinate), which was willing to recognize brain death under certain circumstances, and more conservative ultra-Orthodox circles, who opposed in principle adopting a definition of brain death. The hope was that anchoring the agreement in law would encourage the rabbis of the radical ultra-Orthodox faction to agree to the determination of death and that ultimately a larger segment of the public would be persuaded to sign donor cards. This hope was not unfounded because it reflects a sociological understanding of the system of secularity and religiosity in Israel: obtaining the stricter seal of kashrut was supposed to resolve the religious entanglement that influences the broad public – religious and secular – and prevent religion from serving as a grounds to refuse to donate organs.

The Brain-Respiratory Death Law is to a large extent a song of praise to medical diagnostic technologies, but enjoying the benefits of that technology requires trust in its overseers and operators. That is largely the point: the technology cannot bridge over a gap of mistrust between the sides. Section 8 of the law attests to that. The section discusses informing the family of the death, but it is not clear what that means as far as the determination of death itself. The section establishes different kinds of death and permissions for death, and its convoluted and vague wording is a clear example of the politicization of the issue of brain death.

In fact, it offers two definitions of death, which lead to two sets of interpretation and action: a medical definition and a personal–family definition. Of course, these two definitions may be congruent with each other, but when they are not, the personal–family definition prevails. Section 8d says explicitly:

> Despite the language of this law, whereas brain-respiratory death is determined and this determination opposes the religion or worldview of the patient according to information received from their family, the patient shall not be disconnected from the respirator nor will treatment that directly supports the respiratory therapy be stopped until the heart stops working.

In others words, not only consent to donate but the very definition of death – supposedly a purely scientific matter – is adjudicated by the household economy. Despite the meticulous specification of the means of diagnosis, the establishment of the empowering committee, and the agreement over determination of death (cessation of brainstem activity) – despite all of that, the law actually leads to the entropy of the concept of death, which is to say to disorder in the conceptual sphere of death. This is expressed by the obscurity of the identity of the person who decides about the death, and in granting the power to determine death to a number of parties who may have conflicting considerations. Section 8 actually makes it possible to neutralize the whole law. Even when the determination of death is anchored in law and supposedly there is nothing to prevent deciding on the matter, the final decision remains with the family, with their system of beliefs and opinions and their religious, ethnic, and class affiliations. This means that the ultimate decision on the determination of death is transferred from the civil sphere to the private sphere, in a way that is consistent with the individualization and privatization processes of the organ economy.

The anchoring of the definition of death in the law further emphasized the fact that that definition is a political issue and not a simple declaration of the very fact of death. Like other regulation mechanisms that characterize the political culture of religion and state in Israel, this package deal was mainly a political maneuver, in which separate ethical issues were mixed together in a single political pot. Therefore, the Brain-Respiratory Death Law is different from parallel laws in other countries, both in its definition of death and in the way of determining death.

Four main characteristics distinguish the Israeli law from laws and regulations in other countries. First, its hyphenated title – the Brain-Respiratory Death Law – already indicates that the definition of death in Israel differs from the accepted medical definition in the world, "brain death." The Israeli law contains, in addition to the neurological aspect, the aerobic aspect as well. In fact, death of the brainstem is not presented as an independent criterion but as a sign of the cessation of independent respiratory functioning – like in the Chief Rabbinate's declaration from 1986. Second, section 8 of the law further restricts the medical authority and allows not only the person themselves (through preliminary instructions) but also their family to oppose the declaration of brain death and demand their continued treatment until the determination of cardiac death. This means physicians are required to continue giving life-saving treatment to a person who according to medical criteria is already a cadaver. Third, the law establishes a protocol of the required tests to determine brain-respiratory death, including clinical and instrumental tests, and does not leave the decision to the doctors. This means forcing work procedures on the medical profession and especially on a developing and changing science. Fourth, the law requires establishing an authorization and monitoring committee with equal representation of the Chief Rabbinate and the Medical Association – three representatives each.

Paradoxically, it was precisely the attempt to follow the rules of liberal ethics that led to a legislative process that is a hybrid creature in two senses: first, it hybridized two issues that elsewhere were carefully separated. Second, the Brain-Respiratory Death Law is itself a hybrid of scientific, political, religious, and medical considerations. The goals of combining the two laws were supposed to be achieved in a sort of carefully considered act of legislation: on the one hand, the Transplant Law is similar to parallel laws in the world. It closed the loopholes concerning organ trafficking and, in fact, was intended to return Israel to the bosom of orderly countries that operate according to the accepted bioethical framework. On the other hand, the Brain-Respiratory Death Law put an end to the halachic debate over the definition of brain death.

The anticipated increase in donations from the deceased following this law was supposed to extract Israel from its position at the bottom of the ranking of organ donations from the deceased in the developed countries. It could have also justified toughening the policy forbidding organ trafficking because the Israeli organ economy was supposed to become self-sufficient. However, the Brain-Respiratory Death Law did not manage to achieve the hoped-for agreement, and the opponents of the determination of brain death remained unyielding. Furthermore, in the first two or three years after the law went into effect, the rate of cases of brain death actually dropped because not all hospitals had the required medical equipment to fully diagnose it according to the protocol prescribed by the law.

Two and a half years after the laws passed, at the end of 2010, Avi Cohen, the former captain of the Israeli soccer team, was injured in a motorcycle accident. Cohen, who was wearing an unsafe helmet, sustained a fatal head injury and was taken to Ichilov Hospital in Tel Aviv. His condition deteriorated, and eight days later, he entered the condition of brain death. Cohen, who according to media reports carried a donor card, became upon his death a candidate for organ donation. After his brain death was determined, a team from the National Transplant Center approached Cohen's family asking for permission to disconnect him from the life-support machines and donate his organs. The family agreed and even received the approval of the Chief Rabbi of Israel, Shlomo Amar. But after further consultation, the family retracted and did not let their dear one be disconnected from life support until his heart stopped nine hours later. The press reported a group of yeshiva students from the Braslav Hasidic sect headed by Rabbi Berland had come to the hospital to persuade the family not to disconnect Cohen from the machines (Misgav 2010). Likewise, a newly religious former soccer player called the family while they were filling the consent forms to donate and convinced them not to donate his organs. Avi Cohen's son said in an interview with Yedioth Ahronoth:

> After the doctors talked to us we gathered in the meeting room next to the ICU. Mom said she did not want them to cut Dad and take him apart. She wanted him whole and beautiful as he was in his life. Suddenly there was a deep silence in the room and at that moment we all understood that it was not we who would determine his fate, but that God would in his own way [...] Even if we thought we must honor Dad's wishes, to donate his organs, at that moment of special silence we all understood that it is only God in heaven who gives and takes. At that moment I saw the color come back to everyone's pale faces, as if the burden that was oppressing us disappeared. [...] It is true that father had signed an Adi card and we didn't know, but we couldn't bear to think about the knife cutting him. If I know my Dad, if he could have said last words they would have been: 'Tamir, give the okay to donate my organs and go back to England to do what you need to do.' But [...] it was hard for us to deal with everything at the same time. I had to focus on this new reality that landed on me. [...] During that week I met hundreds of rabbis and smart people. Everyone advised us what to do. I was very confused. One thing was clear to us all at that moment in the meeting room: as long as his heart is beating, we are not disconnecting Father from the machines
>
> (Scheinman and Meidan 2011)

The confusion, the fear, the doubts about brain death, and the fear to donate organs – all are understandable under the difficult circumstances. These feelings are only natural in the terrible situation where the determination of death is incongruous with what the eye sees – because it is not a cold death, with a still and stiff body. In case of brain death, the heart is still beating, the chest is still moving up and down, and the body temperature is maintained by the blood flow. Brain death does not have the resoluteness and the certainty, of death as we perceive it. But contrary to the intention at the basis of the package deal, the involvement of the religious figures in the case of the late Avi Cohen, from the Chief Rabbi to the Berland students, did not help relieve the concerns but actually contributed to the confusion and uncertainty that were already nagging at the family.

The Avi Cohen case is not alone. A few years earlier, chief Rabbi Israel Lau interfered and prevented the donation of the organs of a girl who was brain dead. In 2009, Deputy Health Minister Yaakov Litzman came to Schneider Hospital in Petah Tikva, a few months after taking office, to stand with the parents of a girl who was brain dead and support their decision not to disconnect her from the respirator and life-support machines. In 2014, at Hadassah Hospital in Jerusalem, there was an attempt to train rabbis and influencers from the ultra-Orthodox community so that they would accompany families in cases of brain death and help them make the decision to donate organs. The attempt was cut short at the outset and the entire project was canceled following the opposition of rabbis and heads of the haredi community (Heller 2015). These cases indicate the failure of the concept behind the legislation of the two laws. They show precisely the politicization of the association between brain death and organ transplantation instead of its translation into questions of medical ethics. And, once science and ethics become politicized, it is hard to control the process or determine which agents are allowed to be involved in it.

The Brain-Respiratory Death Law was supposed to conform with the halachic definition of death. But the law, as argued above, was to a large extent another link in the chain of dispute. In fact, the definition of brain-respiratory death persuaded those who needed no persuading. Mainstream Orthodox rabbis did not need the law in order to adopt the compromise proposed by the Chief Rabbinate more than 20 years earlier; Whereas ultra-Orthodox rabbis, whether from the Lithuanian or Hasidic circles, rejected it because of their refusal to recognize death when the heart continues to beat, and perhaps also because of their ingrained suspicion toward the medical establishment. The two laws passed together in 2008 did not reduce the public dispute but actually highlighted the competition between the rabbinical and medical establishments, and the struggle between them over control of the mediation and regulation of end of life. The ongoing dispute over the determination of brain death led to the collapse of the boundaries between science and ethics and their intertwining, with doctors and rabbis remaining players of equal status in the public sphere of the organ economy.

The question of the association between brain death and organ donation remained, after all the discussions and compromises, an open question. The package deal was supposed to blunt the dispute over the definition of death and establish, at least seemingly, a local version of the dead donor rule, in a way that would anchor the separation between death as a scientific issue and donation as an ethical issue. The legislation process was supposed to express the consent achieved in the framework of the law between the medical establishment and the rabbinic establishment and channel the dispute into the format of procedure, a local committee, and a professional question. The failure of the deal brought the question of the connection between brain death and organ donation back into the public sphere so that anyone who had an interest in it was de facto invited to enter the ring. Therefore, numerous parties are stirring the pot in an attempt to establish the nature of the association between the two. The ethical, personal, and familial question concerning organ donation was, therefore, translated into the language of the local political culture, characterized by tension between religion and state, and out of the ruins of the agreements that were supposed to regulate the scientific–ethical mechanism of the dead donor rule arose new political arrangements.

Ironically, the public reverberation of the Avi Cohen affair led to a record number of deceased organ donations the following month: that month, organs were transplanted in 27 patients. A spokesperson for the National Transplant Center said the Avi Cohen affair helped raise awareness of the importance of organ donation:

The publicity given to the matter contributed to a deeper understanding of the brain death issue and its consequences. Most of the families of the deceased comprehended the finality of brain death. In every conversation with a family the issue of respiratory brain death came up with a reference to Avi Cohen's death.

(Gal 2011)

The behavior pattern of Avi Cohen's nonreligious family is an interesting case of the connection between religion and secularity in Israel. Among other things, it appears that secularity disappears when it comes to the beginning and end of life rituals. According to the Gutman Report by the Israel Democracy Institute, on matters of birth and death, many Israelis seek the kashrut seal of the Orthodox stream and follow ancient traditions of lifecycle rites (Kessar-Sugerman and Arian 2011). Many secular Israelis, at the last moments of their or their family members' lives, fear death and often seek an answer to their distress precisely among the religiously strict.

In these situations, religion serves as an agent for crystallizing Israeli identity as an identity with a salient Jewish-religious component. For the Cohen family, religion served as an ideological envelope that provided legitimacy to refusal to donate organs, a refusal that to a large extent came from the fears and uncertainty surrounding the difficult circumstances. This envelope merged science and ethics into a single open question. Nonetheless, no hasty conclusions should be drawn as to the impact of the association between religion and state in Israel on the willingness to donate organs. The tension between the religious and the secular over the issues of brain death and organ donation is not the reason for the failure of the package deal, but rather its outcome. One might say that the political culture of the religion–state relationship in Israel is the lightning rod of the storm of the failure of the package deal and the unresolved internal contradictions surrounding the question of the relationship between brain death and organ donation.

The failure of the Western bioethical concept concerning the Brain-Respiratory Death Law and the Organ Transplantation Law leads to three main conclusions. First, the Israeli legislator's attempt to defuse the tensions surrounding the determination of the moment of death and the separation between the scientific (determining death) and the ethical (organ donation) did not succeed and led to increased politicization of the connection between them. Second, the politicization of that connection was translated into the question of relations between religious and secular and became integrated in a culture where those tensions are managed through compromise, delay of decisions, and creating a status quo. As a matter of fact, the dispute over brain death and organ donation became synonymous with the conflict between religious and secular even before the legislation in 2008 (Boas 2009). Third, even after the legislation, the problem was not solved, and the parties adopted positions that were not necessarily in the public interest. Despite the preliminary agreements, the Orthodox establishment refused to support the determination of brain death, and as a result, the medical establishment, as we shall see forthwith, took measures that exceeded the accepted norms of medical ethics. The public interest, therefore, collapsed into tribalism.

The victory of politics and defeat of ethics

The failure of the package deal, in which both the Brain-Respiratory Death Law and the Organ Transplantation Law were passed together, led to a radicalization of the politicization of the connection between the two. The processes after 2008 are mainly an expression of a power struggle between the sides. In 2012, four years after the compromise deal and the chief legislation in the Knesset, the rabbinate sought to establish a body that would provide guidance and consultation to families on the determination of brain death at the moment of truth. This idea, which ultimately did not materialize, joined other efforts to constitute rabbinic supervision over the determination of death – the most noteworthy among them establishing the religious donor card "Bilvavi" (in my heart). The card was supposed to guarantee that organs were donated after determining brain death following the procedure prescribed by the law – that is, using the required instruments, following the medical protocol that was established, and in accordance with the patient's belief and the family's wishes. The "Bilvavi" card was supposed to serve as the equivalent of the Adi card in the religious sector and thereby could undermine the chief legislation with its overall civil jurisdiction. It could have also undermined trust in the medical profession, which is at the basis of the Brain-Respiratory Death Law. This means that the Chief Rabbinate largely withdrew from its consent to the definition of brain-respiratory death.

To deal with the issues surrounding the existence of two different donor cards, efforts were renewed to bridge between the medical and rabbinic professions. The stumbling block was, as always, the suspicion of rabbinical circles toward the protocol of determining brain death. As a result, a new Adi card was issued, including contact information for rabbinical support. Like the 2008 package deal, the renewed card expresses a compromise between the sides. This compromise allows rabbinic supervision of the determination of death by ratifying medical records, creating joint committees of rabbis and doctors, and training rabbis to accompany families concerning the halachic aspects of determining death. The renewed Adi card includes religious motives, such as the quote from the Mishnah "Whoever saves one life is as if they saved the whole world." It emphasizes the centrality of the family in the decision to donate organs, as well as its right to consult "a rabbi who was qualified and trained in the halachic aspects, who carries a card signed by the Chief Rabbinate of Israel and the Health Ministry," or "a qualified person from another religion," or a doctor, to receive an additional medical opinion. This card, therefore, gives extra force to the religious envelope concerning the routes of organs from one body to another.

The renewed card, which was issued beginning in 2018, expresses yet more forcefully that the question of death is a political rather than a scientific issue. At the center of the dispute was the question of the relative weight of physicians' discretion in determining death. It is an old debate and it had already come up in the Sadgat affair; however, the technology had since improved and new knowledge was gained about the definition of death. The stricter rabbis demanded that the determination of death relies on an objective measurement with instruments, whereas the physicians sought to preserve the status of their professional judgment in determining death. At any rate, once the new card was issued, central rabbis issued a call to sign the card out of a commitment that the determination of death would be made based on an objective examination with instruments. Rabbi Menachem Burstein, head of the Puah Institute (Family Fertility Medicine & Halacha), explained:

> The concern was that the doctor did not manage to 100% diagnose death and therefore we refrained from calling [to sign the Adi card] until it was proved by instruments that the person was really dead. Today, with the introduction of the instruments, we agreed to join forces.
>
> (Ohana 2018)

For the moment, it does not look as if the renewal of the Adi card will manage to motivate the ultra-Orthodox population to sign the card. In any case, once the renewed card was issued, the Bilvavi card was canceled.

This attempt to bridge between the sides indicates a return to the compromise-based consensus model. It is really an attempt to achieve a new package deal that ties the definition of death with organ donation. But as we shall see forthwith, this time, it involves the principle of priority, which prioritizes Adi card signatories to receive organs. I will now review this latest development in the political economics of organ transplantation in Israel.

The priority principle

Prioritizing donor card holders and actual donors is the most noteworthy reaction to the failure of the package deal. As expected, this was the reaction of the medical profession, which views itself as the representative of secular liberalism, science, and progress. The legal background of the principle of priority is section 9b of the Transplantation Law, which states that the steering committee of the National Transplant Center will advise the Minister of Health concerning policy. The steering committee, initiated by Prof. Jacob Lavee, a cardiologist and heart transplant specialist, a prominent representative of the medical community in the area of transplantation, and a former president of the Israel Society of Transplantation, proposed new regulations that gave priority to donor-card holders. The principle of giving priority is simple: Organ donors (living and relatives of deceased organ donors), donor-card signatories (which is to say, potential donors according to the informed consent model), and their families are prioritized in the queue to receive an organ as well as living organ donors (Lavee 2013, Lavee et al. 2013a).

The priority principle also clearly ties the definition of brain death to organ donation and is further testimony of the common history and politics of the two areas. In Israel, as we have seen, that history and politics are associated with the years-long tension between religious and secular. This is what Prof. Lavee wrote about his struggle to apply the priority principle:

> Despite the legitimate criticism, I fought fiercely for the idea, because I thought it had the potential to provide an adequate response to the common phenomenon in Israel of the 'free riderr:' the numerous people who openly declare they are against organ donation, but are not averse to receiving organs from others when they need them. After long discussions it was decided to accept my proposal, but to stipulate its application on chief legislation by the Knesset; legislation that would add the introduction of the nonmedical criterion of signing an Adi card to the list of medical criteria for allocating organs for transplantation.
>
> (Lavee 2013b)

The "free rider" problem is a known problem in public policy and ethics, in general. But in the collective Israeli imagination, the free rider – the parasite – has additional significance connected to the tension between religious and secular and the question of equality in carrying the burden. Supposedly, priority is given by universal criteria: a citizen who does not sign a donor card – secular, religious, haredi, Jewish, not Jewish – is not prioritized in the queue. But actually that presumption of universality is wrong. First of all, the limited access of disempowered groups might prevent them from signing such a card. As we noted, the same problem characterizes the presumed consent model. Second, priority reflects a concept of an autonomous individual, which does not conform with the haredi public and other communities whose members follow the guidance of their religious or spiritual leaders. Third, the priority principle gives a structural advantage to members of large families and opens the way to strategic behavior aimed at increasing chances of receiving an organ – because card signers and their families are given priority in the queue for transplantation, but they will not necessarily become actual donors. It can even be seen as a kind of inheritance: priority to the family is guaranteed by the very signature on an Adi card, and therefore, signing a donor card is not only for personal benefit but also for the benefit of the entire family, even if its other members do not sign it.[1] Furthermore, this principle has value only as long as its application is not universal because if everyone signed a donor card, priority would mean nothing.

The principle of "you sign, you go up the line" reflects an individualist utilitarian concept, according to which the individual is a rational creature acting on their free will and having all the necessary information to make an informed decision. In other words, it is supposed to reflect the ethical agenda of secular liberal ideology. But actually, granting priority is inconsistent with the liberal ethics of medical ethics: even though the reference unit is the rational individual and the guiding principle is autonomous free will, both the background of the priority policy and the context in which it exists actually emphasize the person's social and cultural affiliation. Unlike in game theory computations, in Israeli society, the boundary lines between the groups for which this step is possible and those for which it is not possible are clearly drawn. Furthermore, ironically, the priority principle actually emphasizes the defeat of ethics and victory of politics when it comes to the connection between brain death and organ transplantation. Medical ethics forbid punishing patients and discriminating between them because of their behavior or lifestyle. A person who smokes, for example, knowingly risks their own health, yet they are still entitled to medical care. The priority principle explicitly violates that rule. It draws a novel policy for the distribution of transplantation organs that digresses from the principle of equal treatment for all, regardless of the patient's positions or behavior. By doing so, it reinforces the particular aspect of organ donation and gives mutual altruism – as it is formulated in the ethics of organ donation – a dimension of membership-club style solidarity.

Providing priority, despite its exceptionalism in the global ethical order of organ donation, has so far been accepted in Israel without notable protest. Perhaps it is the politics of shortage: the scarcity of donors in Israel is perceived as a social problem that requires taking unusual measures. According to this concept, procuring organs for donation is related to social behavior and is a common task of society as a whole. And, it is noteworthy that the social action does not violate medical ethics: priority is only one of many considerations that are not purely medical in determining place on the waiting list for transplantation. It does not mean a revolutionary prevailing of a nonmedical criteria over a medical criteria, but rather the strengthening of the social–ethical dimension in determining the waiting list. Yet, adding "a social worth" criterion to the allocation of organs provoked ethical concerns among bioethicists (Barilan 2014). In a recent study, Elalouf, Pliskin, and Kogut (2020) found that medical criteria are more important to the Israeli public in allocating organs than whether the candidate is registered as potential organ donor. Berzon (2018) introduces other six ethical challenges to the priority model. She concludes that such a model can be fair only in a soft opt-out model where the default mode is to donate organs and, hence, to enjoy the priority points (Berzon 2018). Yet, the gist of the priority points is that they work only if just a section of society abides. If all receive the same bonus points, the advantage evaporates. This simple truism attests even more to the restrictive nature of the priority policy and to its "club membership" underpinning concept.

In fact, when asked laypeople about their ethical concerns about the priority policy, some consider it as antisolidarity and aimed against individuals whose beliefs prevent them from signing on donor cards (Guttman, Ashkenazi, Gesser-Edelsburg and Seidmann 2011). In a later study, researchers review the accumulating ethical concerns vis-à-vis Israeli transplant surgeons and other medical practitioners' views and find the policy ethically and practically problematic. They conclude by indicating that 15 years after its enactment "no dramatic change has occurred" (Guttman, Siegal, Appel-Doron and Bar-On 2020).

Social solidarity and the birth of a new altruistic subject

The struggles described heretofore occur as part of the deceased organ economy, and despite the rise in the rate of donations, the shortage problem remains intact. Indeed, in the first years after passing the two laws in 2008, there was a rise in the rate of organ donations from the deceased (Lavee et al. 2013a), and another rise was seen following the priority policy, but it was not enough to create a self-sufficient organ economy. Meanwhile, those who needed transplants ended up worse off: on the one hand, the disagreement over the definition of brain death made it impossible to get out of the stagnation in the deceased organ economy, and on the other hand, the possibility of the organ trade was blocked.

The biggest change in the organ economy in Israel after passing the transplantation law actually occurred in the living organ economy in a way that yet again emphasizes the politicization of the ethical as part of the tension between secularity and religion. An indication of that transformation can be found in the study I did with my colleagues at the Rabin Medical Center on the impact of the Transplantation Law on living organ donations (Boas Mor, Michowitz, Rozen-Zvi et al. 2015). The study found that after the law went into effect there was a rise in the living organ economy, especially as the result of kidney donations inside the family. The Transplantation Law blocks the possibility of transplantation from questionable sources overseas and criminalizes those involved in organ trading so that those who need kidney transplants increasingly rely on family and relatives in their search for an organ. Therefore, the family became the immediate reservoir for kidney donations. The study also checked living donations from outside of the family and found that after the Transplantation Law was passed the social demographic profile of living donors who are not family members changed: the rate of women among those donors rose, as did the average age, the rate of married people, and the rate of people with higher education. The profile of the average donor who was not a relative changed from a single bachelor with low education and income to an adult with a large family, mainly Jewish religious education and low income (ibid).

These findings were surprising because they indicate a change caused by the Transplantation Law although not in the expected direction. First of all, the law sought to change the deceased organ economy, but the change occurred in the living organ economy. Second, the change indicates a new profile of organ donors. Again, the living donors who are not family members are no longer young single men but heads of large families with religious Jewish education. Therefore, the rise in organ donation from the living donors comes from a rise in donations from a particular social sector: Orthodox Jews.

This trend indicates the creation of a new solidarity that is not based on the civil order but on inner communal commitment feelings, something which can be described as an extended family belonging. This solidarity shapes a new kind of altruism and gives birth to a new altruistic subject. This new form of solidarity, which, in turn, gave birth to a new sort of altruistic living donors, is expressed by the activity of the Matnat Chaim ("gift of life" in Hebrew) organization. Like equivalent organizations in the world, Matnat Chaim matches patients who need kidney transplants with unrelated donors. These are people who learned of the stories of people needing transplants and are willing to donate their kidneys to them without prior acquaintance between them. The organization was founded as part of the global trends in organ economics but developed into a central player in the Israeli organ economy. It was founded in 2009 by Rabbi Yeshayahu Heber, himself a kidney recipient who died of Covid-19 in 2020 while realizing his life's work.

The motivation for its establishment by Rabbi Heber was similar to the motivation behind the Adi Association more than 30 years earlier: the death of a young man who was exhausted by dialysis treatments and could not find a kidney donation to save his life. Both organizations are the result of a private initiative and were established following a difficult experience of the shortage of transplantation organs. Both also brought to Israel the global trend that prevailed at the time: the Adi brought the principles of Western ethics of organ donation as developed at that time – including the model of informed consent on the premise of personal autonomy – as well as the growing awareness of organ donation after death and the importance of carrying a donor card, whereas the Matnat Chaim Association brought the pattern of anonymous donation in the living organ economy organization, known as nondirected living organ donation. However, in Matnat Chaim, a different type of altruistic donation is introduced. The donors can express a set of stipulations and preferences as to the general profile of their potential recipients. Do personal stipulations and preferences disqualify the donations from being considered altruistic?

Embedding the question of altruism in a sociological framing helps in answering this difficult question. On the one hand, Matnat Chaim's donors volunteer to sacrifice one of their kidney for saving the life of an unknown stranger. Undeniably, a noble act that only few are willing to commit. On the other hand, selecting from which sector your potential recipient is from contradicts the ethics of altruism as unconditional giving and is in tension with principles of equality and equity. This paradox can be resolved if we contextualize the donation act and the operation of Matnat Chaim in the political economy matrix developed in this book; as pertaining to the private sphere of organ economy where living organ economy produces a new version of donation ethics that are local and contingent. Matnat Chaim, in this respect, produces an ethics of organ donation that is tied to the features of a religious community.

Indeed, one of the prominent features of Matnat Chaim is its Orthodox Jewish character. The organization's website carries the statement: "All of the activities of Matnat Chaim are subject to Jewish Halacha, the Torah, and Jewish morality, from which the organization draws its sense of mission and religious duty." Beneath the statement are endorsements and praise for living donations from the leading rabbis in the haredi community: Rabbi Shlomo Zalman Auerbach, Rabbi Ovadia Yosef, Rabbi Chaim Kanievsky, and Rabbi Yosef Shalom Eliashiv. The support of the heads of the haredi community for living organ donations was known previously, but only as part of Matnat Chaim was that position harnessed for encouraging donations and a practical solution to the shortage problem. Matnat Chaim is no different in that way from similar associations and organizations in the religious and ultra-Orthodox sectors, who seek to accommodate the use of medical technology to the Halacha and the religious normative framework (Ivry 2013, 2010). The rabbis' support for Matnat Chaim shows that their aversion is not to technology or medicine but to the medicalization of death, as arises from the dispute over brain death (Gross, Lavi and Boas 2019).

Therefore, unlike in the deceased organ economy, in the living organ economy, there is actually a positive correlation between level of religiousness and willingness to donate an organ. Most of the donors as part Matnat Chaim belong to the more conservative Orthodox religious sector. The organization's education and recruitment efforts are focused mainly on the religious public – in Sabbath leaflets distributed at synagogues, advertisements in the religious sector's newspapers, and at initiated meetings. The organization's publications are tailored to the differences between the ultra-Orthodox and modern Orthodox communities. Its reports are written in a religious style, for instance, placing the date according to the Jewish calendar before the secular calendar date. The names of the donors and transplantees appear as in Jewish tradition, with the mother's name (Yitzhak the son of Sarah, for example), for the purpose of prayers for recovery and health; Rabbi Heber himself offered blessings of thanks and prayer for the organization's continued success. According to the organization's reports, from the beginning of its activity until 2022, it managed to recruit more than 1,200 altruistic donors. That is an impressive achievement by any scale, and the National Transplant Center lags very far behind. The dizzying rate of recruiting donors by the organization also overshadows the recruitment of donations from the deceased, and to a certain extent, it dulls the edge of need by dialysis patients, which worsened since the 2008 transplant law.

The success of Matnat Chaim is credited largely to the informal economic infrastructure for solving needs and shortages among the religious community and the ultra-Orthodox, in particular. That system is embodied by the systems of charity and aid funds, which provide support to a public many of whose members live beneath the poverty line. In that framework, donating a kidney to someone in need of one is perceived as a religious duty. Thus, for instance, in 2012, after the organization had managed to recruit dozens of donors, the following appeared in the haredi newspaper Yated Ne'eman:

> People from the outside can hardly believe it, but it's a fact! Many dozens of yeshiva students, women, young and old, have donated kidneys in the past two years, voluntarily, for free, most of them to people they did not know. After Sukkoth the 80th transplant initiated by Matnat Chaim is going to take place. The designated donor is a serious and diligent kolel student, and the candidate for the transplant is the wife of another student from another city, a mother of several little children, who will receive one of his kidneys, without any prior acquaintance between the families [...] Who knows whether your neighbor across the street or the secretary at your health fund have quietly donated a kidney, for the sake of a good deed, and this is a point of credit in these times of heresy and repentance.
>
> (Hevroni 2012)

In February 2016, three and half years after the article in Yated Ne'eman, Feiga Stern reported in the daily secular paper Yedioth Ahronoth on a conference of

Matnat Chaim's donors. "The homogeneity of the conference immediately catches your eye," writes Stern. "Black and crocheted skullcaps, earlocks and head scarves. You could count the uncovered heads on the fingers of one hand. Where are the secular?" (Stern 2016). Similar articles appeared in "Bakehila" and "Hapeles", both newspapers for the haredi public. The publicity in these newspapers provided donation with a normative legitimacy and can expand the circle of potential donors. With the expansion of the circle of donors, it was joined by new sectors, still religiously observant, but beyond the Green Line, especially in small settlements. In an interview with Yedioth Ahronoth, Rabbi Heber referred to the wide representation of settlers among Matnat Chaim's donors:

> I respect and value all sectors, but among the settlers there are more people who are willing to give up their comfort for their values. It is much easier and more comfortable to live in Raanana (Central Israeli city HB) than in a distant settlement far from your work and in a dangerous area. Materially, it is a dubious pleasure to live in a place like Yitzhar (remote settlement HB). From my experience, people who decide to donate a kidney, it is not the first good deed they have done in their lives. These are people who in general do good. We have donors from Har Bracha, Eli, Pedu'el (remote settlements HB). By the way, there are already six donors from Eli. A joke has been going around there recently, that a support group opened in the settlement for people who still have two kidneys.
>
> (Ehrlich 2016)

As mentioned, Matnat Chaim's operational model allows stipulating the donation, undermining the universal approach to which the state authorities are committed. In a document describing the organization's ethical rules, it says:

> The right (and some would say the duty) of a person is to prefer those who are close to them. We do so in countless contexts and organ donation is no different. It is even possible that a certain patient's personal story will touch the heart of a stranger and that stranger will decide to donate a kidney to the patient.

The document goes on:

> When a donor comes to Matnat Chaim and asks to volunteer to donate a kidney, the organization will ask them whether they have references as to the identity of the patient who will receive their kidney. Some prefer to donate a kidney particularly to a young person. Some prefer to donate to a man or to a woman. Some prefer to donate to Jewish patients and some have specifically asked to donate to Arab or Palestinian patients. Some will seek to donate to a patient who takes good care of their health such as avoiding smoking and so on. In addition to those we have come across dozens of other personal preferences, according to each donor's subjective choice. Our working assumption is that the donor's choice by independent measures is a legitimate choice and

is equal to giving charity according to the donor's preference. Such a donation is a "gift of life" (like the name of the organization) and the donor has the right to give their gift, in the form of a functioning kidney, to whomever they choose.

Rabbi Heber explains his view on the stipulation clause:

> Moshe was not willing to donate a kidney to someone who might throw stones at him. That is legitimate to me. He has the right to prefer whoever he wants. Some people tell me, 'I want to donate to a young person,' others say the opposite – 'I want to donate to a person with the least chances to receive a donation.' There are some who want to donate only to Sabbath observers, and some ask to donate to a Jew, without any further stipulation.
>
> (Rat 2014)

The stipulation possibility appears in the questionnaire the candidates are asked to fill, under the title of: "Comments and special requests." In a personal interview, I asked Rabbi Heber whether the very existence of that clause does not encourage stipulations to donation. He said the clause was added to the questionnaire precisely because candidates for donation, having gone through the whole matching process, set terms for the identity of the recipient. He believes these terms are legitimate and seek to match the donation to the lifestyle and belief of the donors – after all, it was that lifestyle that led them to donate organs in the first place. Rabbi Heber added that his approach to the religious sector arose from the fact that he himself belongs to that sector, but he wishes to expand the circle of donors to secular Jews and Arabs. Heber adds that ultimately the donation in the framework of Matnat Chaim shortens the general waiting list for transplants and this helps all patients. Ultimately, the determined claim that the donors have the right to donate according to their worldview emphasizes the problematic transition from the civil sphere to the private sphere in organ donation, and the logic according to which the general good arises from limited altruism means that ultimately particularism becomes universalism.

M., from a farming community in the north, described to me the limits of his altruism: it was important to him for the recipient to be Jewish.

> When I saw the notice in the paper I said to my wife, I have two things I will not compromise over: for there not to be some middleman who makes money on my back, and the second is that I would only donate to a Jew. Since I ascertained the existence of both of those things, I didn't care who I was donating to. If I knew there was someone in the system I trusted and they told me it would be donated to a Jew, I would have preferred that to the situation I'm in now, when the transplantee's family calls me every other week to tell me how much they thank me. I would have happily spared them and myself that experience. It is said in Jewish law that the highest level of charity is that the giver does not know who they're giving to, and the recipient does not know

who they received from. In Israel's system today, if I did that it might have gone to an Arab, and that is not so consistent with my worldview. Therefore I had to ascertain who it was going to and therefore I made an appointment to meet the person who posted the advertisement, and it was important for me that it were only a Jew.

M.'s stipulation, that he would donate an organ only to a Jew, undermines the extent of his altruism and stresses the boundaries of his solidarity. It is more of a communal belonging that his donation results rather than universal altruism as one might expect from anonymous donation. In fact, one can say that it turns the nondirected anonymous donation to something more close of a donation within the extended family.

But what kind of altruism is it? Certainly, sacrificing your own kidney to a person in need you do not know is exceptional good deed and it can be considered altruistic act. And yet, the rather vast space in which the donors, their subjective sets of beliefs and selecting the recipient by religious–national criteria, indicate the rise of a new kind of altruism. The new altruistic subjects execute their altruism as part of their self-realization; their experience of being in the world; and their social, communal, gender, and ethnic affiliations. In doing so, they challenge the existent ethics of living donations and undermine the values of equity and equality in organ allocation. But are these ethical values – that pertain to the public sphere and formal transplantation ethics – are valid in the world of private acts of philanthropy? We accept stipulations by private donors in many areas of philanthropic life, why – goes the argument – that this will be different in people that are willing to sacrifice a vital organ for the sake of a person in need?

When I was matched to one such donor in my last transplant, I felt a mixture of gratitude and uneasiness. The gratitude requires no explanation, but the feeling of uneasiness first came from the fact that I am entitled to such a donation by the mere fact that I belong to the hegemonic Jewish sector. Being preferred to donation over the non-Jewish person who sits next to me in the dialysis ward seems simply unfair and unjust. Unlike the bonus of points, I enjoyed following the priority models and the fact that two of my parents donated me their kidneys, entitlement to donation as a result of my religious identity seemed simply wrong.

Moreover, the extraordinary act of donation from a stranger, I feared, would realize the concerns I heard in my third transplant when I bought a kidney. "He would ask you for more money and would never cease to put guilt on you" said to my friends. Well, he did not. But, in this strange manifestation of someone sacrificing his kidney to save me, the quid-pro-quod part is not clear. What are my obligations toward this act? Certainly, the payback is not in money, but if – as Rabbi Heber asserted – "it's their lifestyle that led them to donate in the first place" and given the stipulation clause, would I be expected to endorse the whole set of the donor's identity which is very far from my own. With stories of Gift of Life's donors were filled with self-praise to them and to their sector, I feared they will garner the donation story to an agenda that I do not identify myself with. Indeed, it is the lifestyle of living in a community which flags the slogan of "All Israel are responsible for each other" which is far from the individualistic and secular sector to which I belong. It is specifically this lifestyle that is missing in my secular urban community which does not yield this volume of nondirected donors. But it is also this lifestyle that is so far from my own. I was afraid that under the circumstances of gratefulness I would be expected to endorse not only the noble act of donation but also a complete way of life that is far from me.

In many ways, the story of Matnat Chaim is a story on communities and their inner solidarity. Seen from that perspective, there is affinity between Matnat Chaim and the priority model. In both, organ donation is acted upon a solidarity which is bounded within a defined community. The priority model benefits individuals who pertain to the sector who can consent to the definition of brain death and hence carry donor cards. Matnat Chaim benefits individuals who are part of the Jewish majority. Both effectively establish organ economies based on a bounded solidarity in the model of a membership club. And, in both, there is a gap between the inclusive rhetoric and the exclusive practice. In the priority principle, the particular solidarity is expressed by the fact that it only includes those who support the definition of brain death and carry a donor card. In Matnat Chaim, the inclusion criteria of who is in with us are more spelled out. The individualization of the donation act in Matnat Chaim allows the volunteer to specifically draw the lines of inclusion and exclusion of their solidarity circle. The ethical concern that nondirected living donations in a deep diverse societies will succumb into discrimination and exclusion is put to the test in the Israeli case.

The history of organ transplants in Israel can be told as the story of a failed civic solidarity that crumbled into sorts of communal-based bounded solidarity. To a large extent, the solidarity exercised in Matnat Chaim is an extension of family solidarity, or an expansion of the concept of relatedness to the circle of the ethnic community. The concepts it uses are family, nation, and community. This, for instance, is what Riki Rath writes in her report:

> To the question whether they would agree to donate a kidney even to a non-Jew, they are hard-pressed to answer. Shapira volunteers to do it for everyone: 'A person says 'I'm willing to give a kidney to my brother or even to my cousin, but not to my neighbor.' I say I'm willing to give to my brother, and my cousin, and to my cousin's cousin, and to my whole nation. So that the boundaries of my family have expanded to my nation [...] I have no problem donating to an Arab either, and that physically my kidney would be transplanted in an Arab, but on condition that someone from the Arab's family would donate a kidney in exchange to a Jew. So I'm willing to risk myself so that ultimately someone from my extended family, which is my nation, will receive life, I don't care if it's by my direct donation or by an indirect donation'.
>
> (Rat 2014)

In the previous chapter, we saw the fluidity of the concept of relatedness in transplantation medicine: from a concept that refers to genetic compatibility, relatedness became a concept in the anthropology of kinship. The fluidity of the relatedness concept also allows the fluidity of the concept of solidarity: with a growing number of potential donors, the possibilities for solidaristic acts of donating an organ increases, and as the Israeli case demonstrates, different types of communal solidarities emerge. Furthermore, the crumbling down of the inclusive civic solidarity executed by the state, into bounded sets of solidarities for different publics, is part of the process of individualization and privatization as defined in Chapter 5. These solidarities can be seen as part of the "do-it-yourself" projects of organ procurement, where the social capital of the patients, their sectoral belonging, religious identity, or attitudes toward the medical establishment determine their entitlement as organ recipients. Instead of embracing-all civic solidarity, processes of privatization produce different solidarities for different publics, tailored to the exact normative measurement of given groups.

Sociologist Pitirim Sorokin, one of the leading researchers of altruism, spoke about "creative altruism." He argues that giving has a contagious nature and, therefore, society should give opportunities for altruistic behavior (Sorokin 2002). As we saw before, Titmuss drew his call to encourage altruism from Sorokin. But in the case of Matnat Chaim, it is not altruism that leads to solidarity, but a bounded solidarity, which is limited to the ethnos or religious belonging, leads to altruism. It is the social structure, the habitus, or "their lifestyles" as Heber asserted, that produces the new altruistic subject of the nondirected donor. Unlike the universal altruism of Emmanuel Levinas or Simon Weil, this new altruism is directed to specific group of people. Indeed, even altruism in the model of Matnat Chaim involves giving without expecting any reward, but it is a giving that is subject to a series of stipulations. It means that the giving by the new altruistic subject is the expression of a worldview, preferences, and defined values. These subjects create, by sacrificing part of their body, the new ethics of the organ economy, an ethics that applies within the boundaries of the donor's personal system of preferences.

In a way, Matnat Chaim and the priority model returned the social worth criterion that was denounced by bioethicists since it was implemented in allocating dialysis machines in the 1960s. In contrast with Matnat Chaim, the priority model is implemented on the allocation of deceased organs and became a feature of deceased organ economy. This makes a big ethical difference: whereas the social worth criterion is legitimate in procuring organs in the private sphere of living organ economy, it cannot be a criterion in the public sphere of deceased organ economy. Civic solidarity can cohabitate with more restricted and bounded solidarity only if it operates on different social registers than the formal state-level organ allocation policy. Civic solidarity must adhere to values of equality and equity, while obtaining organs from living donors is all about particular histories of relatedness that can never be confirmed with formal ethics of equality and equity or public criteria of distributive justice.

From the Sadgat affair in 1968 until the development of the priority model and Matnat Chaim, 41 years later, the Israeli case is characterized by unique patterns: brain death in the years before 2008 and all the more so in the 2008 legislation package, and the politicization of the procurement and distribution of organs for transplantation following legislation, as part of the priority principle and the Gift of Life organization. The local chronicle of transplant medicine portrays Israel as having a unique history. But, this history only emphasized what is concealed and hidden in other bioethical cultures. Controversy over brain death, combatting organ trafficking, disputing the authority of the medical profession – all of this exists elsewhere as well. It is in Israel, however, that the bioethics of transplants is so bluntly infused into biopolitics and the general political culture. Researchers claim that the Israeli case is not necessarily unique when it comes to ethical behavior in the face of advanced medical technologies but is the harbinger of a new ethical order that is taking root the world over (Raz 2018). Following this reading, the politicization of the organ economy in Israel may indicate the crumbling of the general ethical order of the organ economy based on criteria of distributive justice, equality, and anonymous donation to the first person on the waiting list. The cracks in that ethical order were created by the rise of the living organ economy, the expansion of the concept of family, but especially because of the privatization and the individualization of the organ procurement mechanism. That transition, from the public sphere of supplying health resources and public goods, to the private sphere of "do-it-yourself" consumerism and welfare, is not unique to the area of the political economy of organs for donation, but in that world, it receives one of its most extreme and clear expressions.

Note

1   See also Berzon (2018) and Quigley et al. (2012).

References

Barilan, Y. M. (2014). From altruism to altruistic punishment: A criticism on granting priority in the waiting list to donor card holders, *Harefua*, 153(3–4), 223–225. (in Hebrew).

Berzon, C. (2018). Israel's 2008 Organ transplant law: Continued ethical challenges to the priority points model. *Israel Journal of Health Policy Research*, 7(1), 1–12.

Birenbaum-Carmeli, D. (2004). 'Cheaper than a newcomer': On the social production of IVF policy in Israel. *Sociology of Health & Illness*, 26(7), 897–924.

Boas, H. (2009). The struggle over the last minute. *Israeli Sociology*, 11(a), 219–241. (in Hebrew).

Boas, H., Davidovitch, N., Filc, D., Hashiloni-Dolev, Y., & Lavi, S. (eds.). (2018). *Bioethics and Biopolitics in Israel: Socio-Legal, Political and Empirical Aspects*, Cambridge: Cambridge University.

Boas, H., Mor, E., Michowitz, R., Rozen-Zvi, B., & Rahamimov, R. (2015). The impact of the Israeli transplantation law on the socio-demographic profile of living kidney donors. *American Journal of Transplantation*, 15(4), 1076–1080.

Efrat, A. (2013a). The rise and decline of Israel's participation in the global organ trade: Causes and lessons. *Crime, Law and Social Change*, 60(1), 81–105.

Efrat, A. (2013). Combating the kidney commerce: Civil society against organ trafficking in Pakistan and Israel. *British Journal of Criminology*, 53(5), 764–783.

Ehrlich, Y. (2016). Kidney givers. *Yediot Ahronoth.* (in Hebrew).

Elalouf, A., Pliskin, J. S., & Kogut, T. (2020). Attitudes, knowledge, and preferences of the Israeli public regarding the allocation of donor organs for transplantation. *Israel Journal of Health Policy Research,* 9(1), 1–13.

Filc, D. (2011). *Circles of Exclusion: The Politics of Health Care in Israel,* Ithaca: Cornell University Press.

Friedlaender, M. M. 2002. The right to sell or to buy a kidney: Are we failing our patients?. *The Lancet,* 359(9310), 970–975.

Gal, A. (2011). A Record number in organ donations. The Avi cohen affair helped. *Ynet.* (in Hebrew).

Green, Y. (2015). *Organ Transplantation: Legislation, Ruling and Practice.* Tel Aviv: Resling. (in Hebrew).

Gross, S. E., Lavi, S., & Boas, H. (2019). Medicine, technology and religion reconsidered: The case of brain death definition in Israel. *Science Technology and Human Values,* 44, 180–208.

Guttman, N., Ashkenazi, T., Gesser-Edelsburg, A., & Seidmann, V. (2011). Laypeople's ethical concerns about a new Israeli organ transplantation prioritization policy aimed to encourage organ donor registration among the public. *Journal of Health Politics, Policy, and Law,* 36(4), 691–716.

Guttman, N., Siegal, G., Appel-Doron, N., & Bar-On, G. (2020). Promoting organ donation registration with the priority incentive: Israeli transplantation surgeons' and other medical practitioners' views and ethical concerns. *Bioethics,* 34(5), 527–541.

Halevy, A., & Brody, B. (1993). Brain death: reconciling definitions, criteria, and tests. *Annals of Internal Medicine,* 119(6), 519–525.

Halperin, M. 2007. *Determining the Moment of Death: An Anthology,* Jerusalem: Schlesinger Institute for Medical-Halachic Research. (in Hebrew).

Hamdy, S. F. (2006). *Our bodies belong to God: Islam, Medical Science, and Ethical Reasoning in Egyptian Life,* New York: New York University.

Hashiloni-Dolev, Y. (2015). Posthumous reproduction (PHR) in Israel: Policy rationales versus lay people's concerns, a preliminary study. *Culture, Medicine, and Psychiatry,* 39(-4), 634–650.

Heller, M. (2015). Hadassa: Rabbis will not encourage organ donations. *Yeditoth Ahronot.* (in Hebrew).

Hevroni, Y. (2012). On Matnat Chaim and kidneys contrition. *Yated Neeman.* (in Hebrew).

Ivry, T. (2013). Halachic infertility: rabbis, doctors and the struggle over professional boundaries. *Medical Anthropology,* 2(3), 208–226.

Ivry, T. (2010). Kosher medicine and medicalized Halacha: An exploration of triadic relations among Israeli rabbis, doctors, and infertility patients. *American Ethnology,* 37(4), 662–680.

Kessar-Sugerman, A., & Arian, A. (2011). *Israeli Jews: A Profile,* Jerusalem: The Israel Democracy Institute.

Kremer, (2001). *Organ Transplantations,* Tel Aviv: Yedioth Ahronot. p. 113. (in Hebrew).

Lavee, J. (2013). Ethical amendments to the Israeli organ transplant law. *American Journal of Transplantation,* 13(6), 1614.

Lavee, J. (2013b). Justice in organ donations. *Haaretz.* (in Hebrew).

Lavee, J., et al. (2013a). Preliminary marked increase in the national organ donation rate in Israel following implementation of a new organ transplantation law. *American Journal of Transplantation,* 13(3), 780–785.

Levy, T. (2008). The day the first heart recipient fought over his life. *Haaretz.* (in Hebrew).

Lock, M. (2002). *Twice Dead – Organ Transplants The Reinvention of Death in Japan and North America*, Oakland, CA: University of California Press.

Misgav, U. (2010). What did Avi Cohen wanted? *Yedioth Aharonot*. (in Hebrew).

Ohana, L. (2018). Five questions to Rabbi Menachem Burstein. *Yediot Ahronoth*. (in Hebrew).

Quigley, M. et al. (2012). Organ donation and priority points in Israel: An ethical analysis. *Transplantation*, 93(10), 970–973.

Rat, R. (2014). Not signing on donor cards but donate organs. *NRG*. (in Hebrew).

Raz, A. (2018). "Reckless or pioneer? Public health genetics in Israel", in H. Boas, et al. (ed). *Bioethics and Biopolitics in Israel: Socio-Legal, Political and Empirical Aspects*. Cambridge: Cambridge University Press.

Raz, A. E. (2009). *Community Genetics and Genetic Alliances: Eugenics, Carriers Testing, and Networks of Risk*, London & New York: Routledge, 223–239.

Reches, A. (1996). A doctor, not a religious commissioner. *Haaretz*. (in Hebrew).

Scheinman, M., & Meidan, A. (2011). I felt I have to stay strong and not to fall into the tomb ans stay there with my father. *Yeditoth Ahronot*. (in Hebrew).

Siegal, G. (ed) (2005). *Blue and White Bioethics*, Jerusalem: Bialik. (in Hebrew).

Stark Offer, I. (2015). Philosophical justifications for setting criteria of determining the moment of death according to Jewish Law. PhD dissertation submitted to the department of Philosophy, Bar Ilan University, Israel. (in Hebrew).

Stern, P. (2016). Kidneys contrition. *Yediot Ahronoth*. (in Hebrew).

Sorokin, P. (2002) [1954]. *The Ways and Power of Love: Types, Factors, and Techniques of Moral Transformation*, West Conshohocken, PA: Templeton Press.

Teman, E. (2019). The power of the single story: Surrogacy and social media in Israel. *Medical Anthropology*, 38(3), 282–294.

Traubman, T. (2002). Not quite dead. *Haaretz*. (in Hebrew).

Weiler-Pollack, D. (2008). The heartbreak behind the first heart transplant in Israel. *Haaretz*. (in Hebrew).

Epilogue
When the Shortage Ends

A groundbreaking study was published in July 2021, offering a novel method of organ transplantation (Cohen, Partouche, Gurevich et al. 2021). The researchers propose a solution that would revolutionize the world of transplantation. Their solution is twofold: they would solve the problem of the organ shortage by transplanting people with organs from animals (the study used porcine organs), and the rejection problem would be solved by coating the organs with a genetically engineered tissue from human stem cells that do not stimulate rejection. While xenotransplantation, transplantation of organs taken from animals, is not a new idea and has been part of medical research for decades (Cooper, Ekser and Tector 2015), the solution to organ rejection is novel and revolutionary. It creates hybrid transplantable organs: organs from animals coated with human tissues produced from stem cells extracted from placentas. That combination, chimerism in scientific language, is supposed to provide the solution to the two main problems of the world of transplantation: organ shortage and organ rejection.[1]

The report of the successful experiment is an important step in a long, multi-staged and challenging road at the end of which it may be possible to transplant hybrid organs into human beings. Another path for the future of organ transplantation is paved by scientists and experts in engineering and manufacturing artificial organs. In 2019, another team of researchers have successfully printed a heart. Using technologies of genetic editing, the team obtained living tissues from the patient and modified them twice: from fat cells to stem cells and from stem cells to different heart cells and used them to bioprint a human heart (Noor, Shapira, Edri et al. 2019). Similar experiments in 3D bioprinting of tissues and organs are conducted in accelerating frequency in the last decades, with the hope to produce a personalized engineered organ for transplantations (Skylar-Scott, Uzel, Nam et al. 2019, Ravnic, Leberfinger, Koduru et al. 2017).

As these technologies are still in their experimental stage, they provide hope but no actual foreseeable relief for those waiting for organ transplants. Their lives remain as they have been: lengthening waiting lists, a chronic organ shortage, and the search for hope through alternative channels of organ supply. Does the experiment really herald for us, organ recipients, a new horizon?

I would like to cling to hope not only as a source of optimism as someone who has already undergone four transplants and doesn't know what the future holds

DOI: 10.4324/9781003288886-11

but also to conduct, at the conclusion of this book, a thought experiment that will emphasize what this future holds in terms of ethical challenges. On the one hand, how would transplantation medicine look like without organ shortage? Without the burden of searching for an organ and the danger of rejection? On the other hand, would it be a "brave new world"? with even more pressing ethical concerns?

Let's start with an historical perspective: it can be argued that since its inception, transplantation medicine underwent three revolutions. The first occurred in the very breakthrough in the 1950s and 1960s when it was proven that human organs could be transplanted in other bodies as a solution to end-stage diseases and terminal medical conditions. Kidney, heart, pancreas, liver, and lung transplantations developed during that period and marked transplantation as one of the peaks of technological achievement of modern medicine. That revolution was a technological leap forward, but transplantation remained experimental medicine. Transplanted organs were rejected after a short time and transplantation medicine lingered on the boundary between treatment and research for the most part of the 1960s and 1970s. In the early 1980s, the first cocktails were synthesized to treat the rejection problem and the first generation of immunosuppressant medications was introduced. This pharmacological advancement marks the second revolution in transplantation medicine: "the immunosuppressive revolution." With immunosuppressive treatment, transplanted organs had a long lifespan in the host body and transplantation medicine turned into routine medicine. From the 1980s onward, transplantation medicine spread throughout the world not only at centers of medical innovation, and transplants became an accepted and successful solution for numerous patients. That is the background, as described in Chapter 1, of the development of the organ shortage problem. The medical success gave rise to the growing demand for organs and the sharp increase in the number of patients waiting for a transplant.

The third revolution in the world of transplantation is the subject-matter of this book. The rise in alternative channels of organ supply and the growth of a living organ economy undermine the ethical bases of transplantation medicine. That revolution, which can be understood as "the privatization revolution" – turning the search for a transplantation organ into a private and personal challenge for the patient – is the third revolution. Patients in need of an organ, mostly renal patients, use their social capital, networking, and other means that at their disposal to achieve their life-saving organ. As demonstrated in the last chapters of this books, an extended pool, ranging from family members, close friends, and acquaintances, to even complete strangers join the circle of potential living organs. With no need for human-sourced organs, organ economy will surely change. But what will this change entail? Will hybrid or printed organs herald the fourth revolution of this medicine?

I suggest that the answer is a strong positive. The transplantation of hybrid or printed organs will bring with it a bundle of ethical and moral concerns that will surely render the political economy of organ supply totally different from that which is described in this book. The basic conditions of such economy will be different: from human-sourced organs to scientifically produced organs. The main axis that spins the political economy of organ transplantation, the shortage problem, will disappear. What form will the political economy of transplant medicine take when the shortage ends?

More than six decades of transplantation medicine prove a simple truth: the solution of extracting an organ from one person in order to transplant it into another person has not taken root in society.[2] At least not to such an extent that can satisfy the needs of transplantation medicine. Furthermore, organ transplantation technology created states of dependence and inequality between people, between donors and recipients, and between sellers and buyers. The medical success of organ transplantation led the political economy of organ transplantation into dark alleys of commerce and exploitation. The moral pinnacles of donation out of generosity and social solidarity exist of course, and they too are a cultural expression that accompanies transplantation medicine, but unfortunately, they are expressions that may be gratifying but are insufficient to bridge over the widening shortage. What would the political economy and justifications that go with it look like in hybrid or engineered organ medicine? In what follows I will explore the ethical quandaries that may associate each of these future technologies and conclude by referring a future political economy of organ supply

Xenotransplants – transplanting hybrid organs

Raising animals in order to transplant their organs in humans is not the ideal solution, but solving the problem of organ shortage is an accomplishment that cannot be dismissed. Until the time human organs can be grown by genetic engineering from the patient's own cells, organ transplantation will always mean using the organs of one being to save another, and it will always have to provide a moral envelope and ethical justification for the exploitation embodied in the very concept of transplantation medicine. Beyond the medical questions and risks of xenotransplantation, such as, for instance, the spread of pathogens against which the animal is immune to, but humans are not (Fishman 2020), xenotransplantations carry with them a bundle of ethical quandaries (Schicktanz 2012). The very idea of raising animals for transplantation can spark aversion and resistance among certain circles, especially animal-rights activists. This can be countered with the argument that transplanting an animal organ in a human patient is one of the most justified uses of animals by humans. If humanity changes its customs and its attitude towards animals and stops eating meat, using eggs, milk, or other animal products, the leather industry stops existing and the pet world undergoes a radical change, then, if it does exist, the industry of animal husbandry for organ transplants and saving lives is to be the last to pass from the world, if at all.

And it will be an industry. The industry of animal organs for transplantation will be a commercial enterprise and each transplantation organ will have a price. That industry will surely be integrated in the private market with medical oversight and regulation that will assure the competence of the organs that arrive for transplantation. If we adopt the experiment mentioned above as the model for xenotransplantation, then the animal organs will be coated by human placental cells to provide a solution to the rejection risk. Will placental cells, which presently are donated by women after giving birth, also become a commodity?

According to current legislation in the United States and many other countries, the sale of placental cells is illegal. But will the transition to hybrid transplantation organ medicine change the legislation and jurisprudence concerning organ transplantation? That legislation and jurisprudence, as described in this book, seek to regulate organ donation from humans. It is concerned mainly with the questions of consent, compensation, and medical care for the donor. None of that will be relevant anymore once organs no longer come from humans. But what about the tissue coating the organ, which comes from placental cells? Will its sale be permitted? If not, what will the new justifications be for prohibition of such sale? As opposed to any other organ, the placenta is ejected from the body during birth anyway. If the supply of hybrid organs is fully within the private market, why not remunerate the birthing mother in the end as well? On the other hand, will its sale not increase the price of the transplanted organ? Is this not an extreme case of paying for a body product that the body no longer needs, whose donation involves no special effort or risk? The legislation and regulation system will have to readjust itself to the political economy that will arise from hybrid transplantation medicine.

And what about religious or cultural prohibitions? In Judaism and Islam, pigs are considered impure and their eating is forbidden. But the transplantation of porcine heart valves is permitted in Judaism and with certain adjustments in Islam as well (Easterbrook and Madden 2008). The value of saving a life is paramount and outweighs the prohibition of impurity in other life circles. This might be the case with porcine organ transplantation as well. The history of human organ transplantation medicine shows that the main difficulty confronting religious leaders had to do with the definition of brain death and harvesting organs from brain-dead people. That is also the point that caused a crisis of trust toward transplantation medicine among wide circles who are more suspicious toward advanced medical technology to begin with. What will the dispute over brain death look like in an era when cases of brain death no longer serve as potential sources for organ donation? The unbearable experience of the request to donate organs while the family still surrounds their loved one's body – still warm, its chest still rising and falling with the movement of the artificial respirator – and being asked to approve disconnection from the machinery, will pass from the world. It is one of the most difficult scenes that can be imagined and encompasses a terrible drama that cannot be expressed by any word in any lexicon. But when cases of brain death remain merely cases of brain death, with no connection to organ donation, will it be easier to resolve the dispute around them? Will it be easier to resolve the primary ethical concern surrounding that state of death, namely, extending life that is no longer independent of a machine?

"Welcome to the age of bioprinting: where the machines we've built are building bits and pieces of us"[3] – transplanting printed organs

Bioprinting of organs for transplantations is the second technology that attracts hopes and anticipations for ending the shortage problem. Similar to the development of hybrid organs, the conspicuous advantage in printed organs is rendering the ethics of human organ donations redundant. Nonetheless, the use of printed organs stirs another set of ethical concerns. These concerns stem from the fact that printed organs, unlike hybrid or totally human-sourced organs, are manufactured and produced in a process that resembles an industrial process. Another crucial aspect is the convergence with personalized or precision medicine. With bioprinting, tissues or cells are taken from the patient and modified, through genetic editing to stem cells and then to the designated manufactured organs. Looped together, these two aspects raise ethical concerns in three interrelated domains: the very definition of health and illness, commodification, and enhancement.

Currently, a healthy organ for a transplantation is a functioning organ. What is the level of function for an organ to be transplantable? The answer varies. With the advancement of surgery technique and post-operative care, the range of possible organs that can be transplanted expands and now includes "marginal organs" as well. Where the optimal candidate for deceased organ donation is a young male in a state of brain death, in which his organs still preserve their vitality due to artificially operated blood circulation, marginal organs refer to organs taken from either patients after cardiac arrest (where there is no constant supply of oxygenated blood to the organs), or organs taken from persons at old age, or sometime from a constellation of both cases (Tullius, Volk and Neuhaus 2001). These definitions of transplantable organs will change with printed organs. A reference point for a satisfactory level of functioning will no longer be the donor's constitution. It could be expected to function at a higher level. Which level? That of the patient according to his physical traits? Of a young athlete? For example, a terminal cardiac patient waiting today for a heart transplant can hope for "a good enough" heart that will save his or her life. But with printed organs, the expectations could be higher. Based on the patient's genetic makeup, the ethical concern that bioprinting techniques could generate "super" organs.

Health and illness are, indeed, relative concepts. The shifting boundary between definitions of health and illness is bounded in a set of expectations from what medicine can offer and from the ways in which society frames what is health and what is not in terms of ableism and disablism. But with artificially produced organs, health becomes under the manufacturer's warranty. Printed organs will become a commodity to be sold in the market. Since they are produced, and unlike human-sourced organs or to some degree hybrid organs, they have production costs and value. This might turn them into sheer commodities. And commodities, under the neoliberal imperative of consumerism and competitive markets, are always in the frantic race of updating, improving qualities, and marketing new versions. Think of your cellular phones and their updated versions and think of fashion and trends. The term healthy will then be charged with consumerist marketing of what could be the best organ for you. Such a market will seek a wider audience and could imitate the already existent billions dollar markets of aesthetic medicine. The trend of personalized medicine would only thrust this further with commercial bio-tech companies that will promise to tailor an organ especially for you. Will there be a limit? Could a person purchase a manufactured printed organ based on his own genetic makeup that its manufacturer warranty guarantee is for, perhaps, decades? This would be the most valuable possession a person could get. Perhaps at the age of 120 when this person's other organs fail, the inheritors would quarrel over this organ?

Commodification and enhancement are interconnected here. Enhancement is the term to describe the production – through advanced technologies such as genetic editing and engineering or bioprinting – of tissues or organs that enhance the recipient human capabilities above normal levels. The concept of enhancement and its ethical implications are widely discussed in the bioethical literature (Clarke, Savulescu, Coady et al. 2016, Buchman 2011). Opponents to enhancement address it as a contemporary manifestation of the notorious eugenics that stood at the basis of Nazi medicine (Vizcarrondo 2014). Others reject this, referring to a difference between negative and positive eugenics, arguing that enhancement will advance humanity further with the ability to fully exercises their potential and, thus, contribute to their well-being (Savulescu, Sandberg and Kahane 2011, Sparrow 2011 responding). But will printed organs be a radical extension of "anti-aging" procedures? Moreover, with the temptation of wider audience, commercial manufacturers of printed organs may soon leave the intended population of patients waiting for organs in order to save their life as they will not be able to pay the high price of printed organs or that "ordinary" organs will no longer be worth producing.

This is certainly a dystopic future for transplant medicine. Mostly since the definitions of health and illness are always embedded in power relations of inequality between the have and the have-not. Access to health resources is dependent upon class and social status. The fear is that the commodification of non-human sourced and manufactured organs will only exacerbate such inequalities.

However, these future alternatives should not be forsaken for the ethical challenges they pose. Some of them could be met with a regulation and supervision model that will guarantee that the distribution of printed organs will be under the monopoly of public health agencies. They will be distributed according to need in similar fashion that deceased organs are allocated to transplantations today. The technical improvement of printed organs to the stage of enhancement should also be supervised, discussed, and monitored and private attempt to create a market for printed organs can be outlaws. There are other sets of ethical and regulative challenges that printed organs bring about (Vijayavenkataraman, Lu and Fuh 2016). But the promise that these future paths hold for those who die each day waiting for an organ could not be thrown aside. Printed and hybrid organs should be public health resources, to be developed by public funds, and to be in the sole possession of state's health agency as a barrier against commodification.

* * *

Imagining a future world of new technologies of producing organs for transplantations leads us to think on the differences between now and this futuristic medicine. Surely, the transition of the organ transplantation world to a post-humanist world, one that breaks through the boundaries of the human and the non-human and gives birth to a hybridization of human and animal, printed organic organs has its set of moral perils and concerns. Such a future could be easily imagined in gothic terms. But with the right regulation, it would grant end-stage patients with life with no waiting lists, without the fear of repeating rejections, without aggressive lifelong immunosuppressive treatments, and without entering the bundle of, sometimes, impossible relations with the one who gave you the "gift of life." No doubt the future holds exciting possibilities for transplantation medicine that will make everything in this book redundant and irrelevant. I wish.

Notes

1   Another successful experiment in xenotransplantation was reported on October 2021. In this case, the scientists modified the genetic make-up of pigs so that their future generation could provide safe organs for transplantations. See https://www.nytimes.com/2021/10/19/health/kidney-transplant-pig-human.html (accessed October 21st). Just a few months later, on Jan 22, a genetically modified heart was retrieved from a pig and transplanted in a 57 years old patient. See https://www.nytimes.com/2022/01/10/health/heart-transplant-pig-bennett.html?searchResultPosition=1.
2   Apparently, at least for living organ donations, the shortage could be totally eliminated. The volume of people in the waiting lists for kidney transplantations is only but a fraction of parentage from the total populations. In the US, for example, more than 90,000 candidates for kidney transplants are waiting for a transplant (https://optn.transplant.hrsa.gov/data/view-data-reports/national-data/# accessed 1 Jan 2022). With a population of 330 million, there are – theoretically – more than 3,300 possible candidates as organ donor for a single patient. This ratio should have sufficed to satisfy the demand for kidney transplant. The fact that 90,000 people wait 3–5 years in dialysis attests to the fact that the practice of organ donation is far from being an acceptable norm. The situation is no different in other countries. Organ donation does not enjoy a wide legitimization basis.
3   A sentence appearing in the online platform of the oxford dictionary definition for bioprinting. https://www.lexico.com/definition/bioprinting (accessed Jan. 2nd).

References

Buchanan, A. E. (2011). *Beyond Humanity?: The Ethics of Biomedical Enhancement*, Oxford: Oxford University Press.

Clarke, S., Savulescu, J., Coady, C. A. J. et al. (eds.). (2016). *The Ethics of Human Enhancement: Understanding the Debate*, Oxford: Oxford University Press.

Cohen, S., Partouche, S., Gurevich, M. et al. (2021). Generation of vascular chimerism within donor organs. *Scientific Reports*, 11(1), 1–15.

Cooper, D. K., Ekser, B., & Tector, A. J. (2015). A brief history of clinical xenotransplantation. *International Journal of Surgery*, 23, 205–210.

Easterbrook, C., & Maddern, G. (2008). Porcine and bovine surgical products: Jewish, Muslim, and Hindu perspectives. *Archives of Surgery*, 143(4), 366–370.

Fishman, J. A. (2020). Prevention of infection in xenotransplantation: Designated pathogen-free swine in the safety equation. *Xenotransplantation*, 27(3), e12595.

Noor, N., Shapira, A., Edri, R. et al. (2019). 3D printing of personalized thick and perfusable cardiac patches and hearts. *Advanced Science*, 6(11), 1900344.

Ravnic, D. J., Leberfinger, A. N., Koduru, S. V. et al. (2017). Transplantation of bioprinted tissues and organs: Technical and clinical challenges and future perspectives. *Annals of Surgery*, 266(1), 48–58.

Savulescu, J., Sandberg, A., & Kahane, G. (2011). Well-Being and enhancement. In Savulescu, J. Ter Meulen, R & Kahane, G (eds), *Enhancing human capacities*, Oxfordshire: Blackwell publishing, 1–18.

Schicktanz, S. (2012). "Xenotransplantation", in R. Chadwick (ed). *Encyclopedia of Applied Ethics*, Second Edition, volume 4. San Diego: Academic Press. pp. 565–574.

Skylar-Scott, M. A., Uzel, S. G., Nam, L. L. et al. (2019). Biomanufacturing of organ-specific tissues with high cellular density and embedded vascular channels. *Science Advances*, 5(9), eaaw2459.

Sparrow, R. (2011). A not-so-new eugenics: Harris and Savulescu on human enhancement. *The Hastings Center Report*, 41(1), 32–42.

Tullius, S. G., Volk, H. D., & Neuhaus, P. (2001). Transplantation of organs from marginal donors1. *Transplantation*, 72(8), 1341–1349.

Vijayavenkataraman, S., Lu, W. F., & Fuh, J. Y. H. (2016). 3D bioprinting–an ethical, legal and social aspects (ELSA) framework. *Bioprinting*, 1, 11–21.

Vizcarrondo, F. E. (2014). Human enhancement: The new eugenics. *The Linacre Quarterly*, 81(3), 239–243.

Index

Note: **Bold** page numbers refer to tables; *italic* page numbers refer to figures and page numbers followed by "n" denote endnotes.

For Product Safety Concerns and Information please contact our EU
representative GPSR@taylorandfrancis.com
Taylor & Francis Verlag GmbH, Kaufingerstraße 24, 80331 München, Germany